CW01260901

a colour illustrated atlas

Gastroenterology in the Elderly

a colour illustrated atlas

Gastroenterology in the Elderly

Volume 1

Edited by   A G Vallon   J R Armengol Miro
Consultant Physician   Associate Professor
Crawley Hospital   Universidad Autonoma Barcelona
Crawley   Barcelona
West Sussex   Spain.
UK.

Lilly

**Presented as a service to medical education
by Eli Lilly & Company Limited**

This book comprises volume 1 of a 3 volume series entitled
Gastroenterology and the Elderly: a colour illustrated atlas

Any product mentioned in this book should be used in accordance with the prescribing information prepared by the manufacturers. No claim or endorsement is made for any drug or compound presently under clinical investigation.

This book represents the findings of its authors and its contents do not necessarily reflect the opinion of Eli Lilly & Company Limited.

Copyright © 1988 by Science Press Limited
Phillipp House, 20 Chancellor's Street
Hammersmith Riverside
London W6 9RL

All rights reserved. No part of this publication may be reproduced, stored in a retrieval system, or transmitted in any form or by any means electronic, mechanical, photocopying, recording or otherwise without prior written permission of the publishers.

British Library Cataloguing in Publication Data

Gastroenterology in the elderly

1. Old persons.   Gastrointestinal tract Diseases.
I. Vallon, A.G.
II Armengol Miro J.R.

618.97'633
ISBN 1-870026-35-7

Designed by Robin Dodd FCSD
Linework by Lynda Payne
Printed in Italy by Imago Publishing Limited
Typeset by Informat Computer Communications Limited

Contents

PAGE 8 Introduction *A G Vallon*

PAGE 20 Diseases of the mouth *P L Golding*

PAGE 36 Oesophageal disease and the elderly *A S Mee*

PAGE 58 Gastro-duodenal disease in the elderly *R W Stockbrügger*

PAGE 78 Index

Contributors

A G Vallon
Consultant Physician
Crawley Hospital
Crawley
West Sussex
UK

J R Armengol Miro
Associate Professor
Universidad Autonoma Barcelona
Barcelona
SPAIN

P L Golding
Consultant Physician
Department of Gastroenterology
Queen Alexandra Hospital
Cosham
Hampshire
UK

A S Mee
Consultant Physician
and Gastroenterologist
Battle Hospital
Reading
Berkshire
UK

R W Stockbrügger
Associate Professor and
Medical Director
Marbachtalklink
Der Landesversicherungsanstalt
Oldenburg-Bremen
Bad Kissingen
FRG

Introduction
A G Vallon

Figure 1.1
Population changes since 1850.

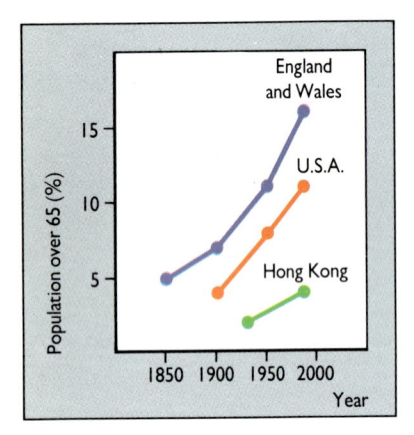

Ageing and population growth

The over-65s form just under 16% of the population of England and Wales, a similar proportion to that found in most other countries of north-western Europe. In the United States, where there is still net immigration and population growth, the over-65s form just under 12% of the population, although it is projected that within the next 50 years the proportion of the elderly within the population of the United States will rise to around 16%. In the newly industrialized countries of the Far East (for example, Hong Kong) the population profile is similar to that of England 100 years ago when only 5% of the population were elderly. Here net immigration of young workers coincides with a very high birth rate to produce a young population (Figure 1.1).

The ageing of our population during the last 100 years or so has been positively affected by the improvement in living standards and, to a lesser degree, public health measures. There has been a tenfold reduction in the infant mortality rate, and the vast majority of children born nowadays can expect to survive to become young adults. Major diseases such as smallpox, typhus, typhoid fever, scarlet fever, rheumatic fever and diphtheria have to a large extent been eradicated, due to better nutrition, improved sewerage and immunization. The introduction of sulphonamides in the 1930's, antibiotics and anti-tuberculous therapy in the 1940's and 1950's largely contributed to the elimination of severe bacterial diseases which used to kill young adults.

Despite all these improvements in health, the longevity of man has altered very little. In 1851 a man who had survived to 65 could expect to live for a further 10 years, and in 1988 his life expectancy has increased by a further 2 years. Gerontologists estimate that life span, the maximum obtainable age by man, is 85 years, so that even if all disease were eradicated we could not anticipate a massive improvement in life expectancy.

The proportion of the elderly to the rest of the population is not expected to increase further in the U.K. (Figure 1.2). Thus the dire predictions that there will not be sufficient workers in 30 years time to generate the wealth to pay for the pensions of the present working population when they themselves become pensioners are unjustified. The total number of pensioners as a proportion of the population will not change substantially, however, there will be a change in the profile of the ages of the elderly. It is projected that there will be a fall in number of the age group 65–74, whilst those aged over 75 will increase by 20% and those aged over 85 will increase by 40%, compared with today's figures. This has enormous implications for those people providing health and social care. It is the very old who are the most likely to be users of health care and who occupy many hospital beds (Figure 1.3).

Ageing and treatment advances

More than half of the acute medical and surgical beds in most district hospitals are occupied at any one time by people over the age of 65. Whilst cancer in children and young adults rightly attracts enormous attention, the majority of patients in hospital for cancer treatment are over 65. Although they comprise less

	1986	2001
Total population (millions)	50.1	52.2
Total 65+	7.8 (15.5%)	8.2 (15.7%)
65–74 years	4.5 (8.9%)	4.2 (8.1%)
75+	3.3 (6.6%)	4.0 (7.6%)
85+	0.64 (1.3%)	1.05 (2%)

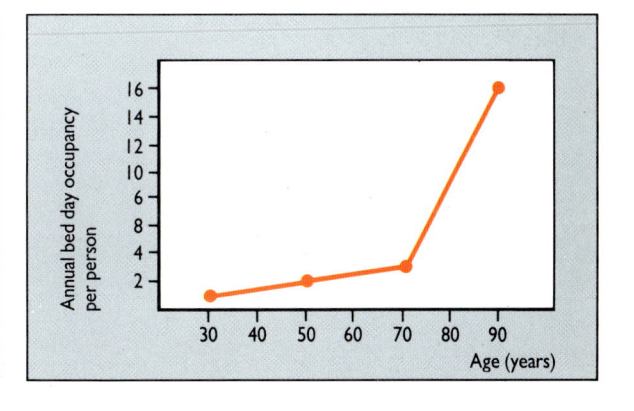

Figure 1.2
Projected population changes in England and Wales 1986–2001.

Figure 1.3
Hospital activity in England and Wales. Bed occupancy according to age.

than one-sixth of the total population of this country they are responsible for almost half the drugs prescribed by physicians. Many elderly people receive prescriptions for many different preparations at the same time because of their multiple ailments. As the proportion of the very elderly increases it is likely that more medical resources will be needed for them.

Only in the last 40 to 50 years has it become widely recognized by doctors that old people become immobile, confused, have falls and develop incontinence because of treatable physical illness and not necessarily because of senility. The old benefit enormously from many of the recent major advances in medical technology. It is commonplace for an otherwise fit 80-year-old who has been rendered disabled by osteoarthritis of the hip to be rejuvenated by hip replacement. Fifteen years ago in England, cardiac surgery was restricted to the under 60s in many cardiac centres. Nowadays a 75-year-old whose sporting activity is severe-

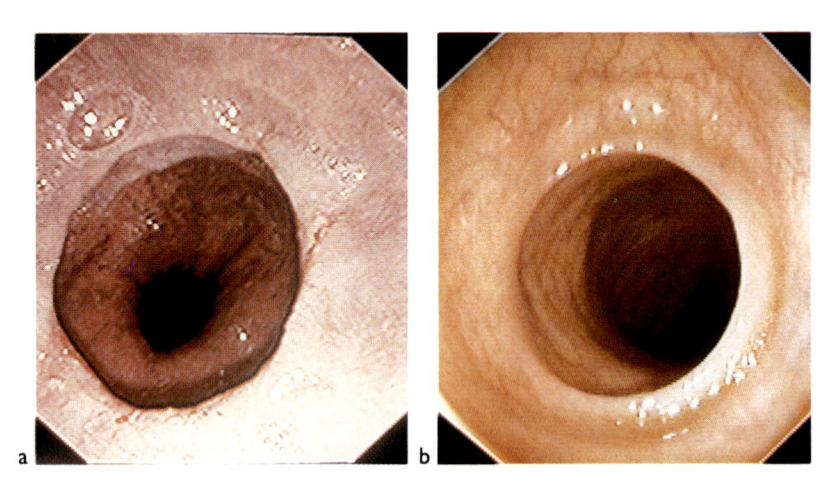

Figure 1.4
Endoscopic views of:
a Normal oesophago-gastric junction. The oesophagus is lined by squamous epithelium producing a white sheen. The stomach is lined by columnar epithelium which shows as deep pink.
b The sigmoid colon showing a normal vascular pattern.
c The transverse colon showing typically pronounced triangular haustral folds and a normal vascular pattern.

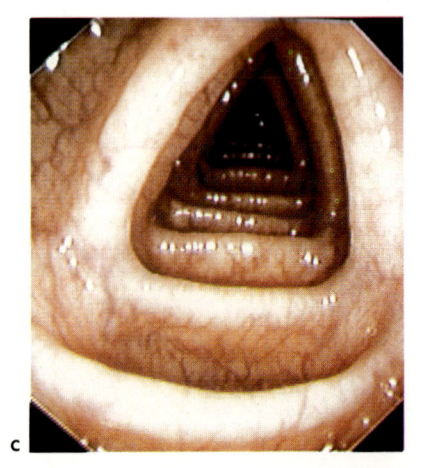

ly limited by angina can be referred for, and expect to receive, coronary artery bypass surgery. The improvements in our understanding of gastrointestinal disease and the technical advances of the last 20 years have been particularly beneficial to elderly people. Like geriatric medicine, gastroenterology is a relatively young specialty. Major advances in gastroenterology during the last 20 years have coincided with the availability of highly flexible, easily manipulated fibre-optic endoscopes which allow visualization of the gastrointestinal tract. (Figure 1.4a to c).

The advent of endoscopy
Before the availability of endoscopes, access to the gastrointestinal tract, was very limited. The rigid and semi-rigid early endoscopes were difficult to use and the views obtained were often poor. The procedures were unpleasant and often painful for the patient and radiology using barium was really the only reliable investigation available for the colon and stomach.

Modern fibre-optic endoscopy is very well tolerated by the patient. In most elderly patients provided the procedure is explained beforehand, endoscopy can be performed with very little sedation. Usually a small dose of pethidine, 25 mg given intravenously, combined with 5 mg of diazepam, will produce relaxation without any respiratory depression. The only major contraindications to upper gastrointestinal endoscopy are the presence of a Zenker's diverticulum or respiratory failure. The technique of intubation can be a little more difficult in the elderly because of the presence of disease of the cervical vertebrae, and it is important that endoscopy is only performed by or under the supervision of experienced endoscopists. As well as being an excellent diagnostic and therapeutic tool, fibre-optic endoscopy has allowed the study of the process of ageing of the stomach and small intestine, and the very accurate assessment of the efficacy of new drugs.

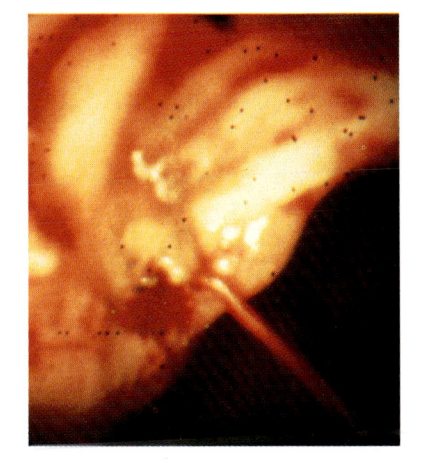

Figure 1.5
Arterial bleeding from a vessel in the base of a gastric ulcer.

H$_2$ receptor antagonists (H$_2$ blockers)
One group of drugs which has had a dramatic effect on the natural history of a disease has been the H$_2$ receptor antagonists in peptic ulcer disease. In the early 1970's most general surgeons' operating lists had one or more patients undergoing surgery for treatment of a peptic ulcer. Nowadays it is rare for such operations to be performed, except in emergencies such as gastrointestinal bleeding (Figure 1.5) or ulcer perforation. Cimetidine, the first of the H$_2$ blockers to be released commercially, came into general use in 1977. Its impact was emphasized by the accurate

demonstration by endoscopy of duodenal ulcer healing, something which would not have been possible if only barium studies had been available (Figure 1.6a to c).

Ageing of cells

There is little evidence that ageing of the cells of the gastrointestinal tract produces symptoms or disease, except perhaps in the oesophagus where the condition of presbyoesophagus (old age oesophagus) is recognized. Many very elderly people will have impaired or absent peristalsis of the oesophagus. Rarely, even when peristalsis is absent, does it seem to cause significant symptoms.

Dietary factors

Many of the diseases of the gastrointestinal tract in old people may be the result of many years of dietary abuse. It is probable

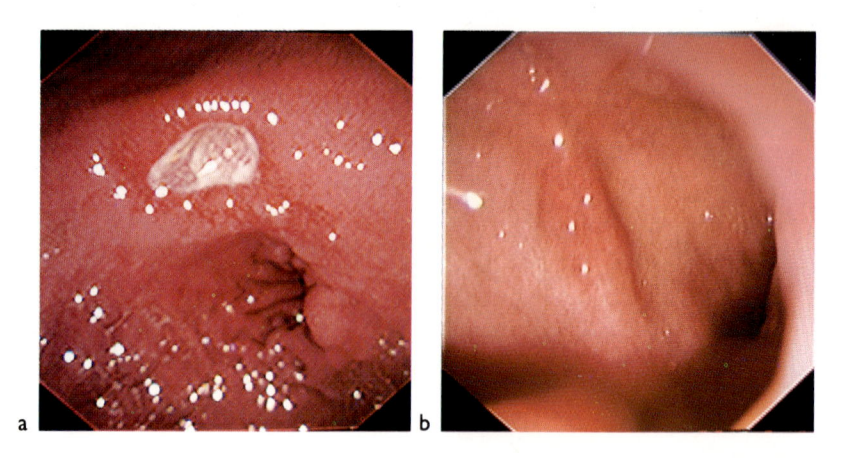

Figure 1.6
a Duodenal ulcer.
b Site of healed duodenal ulcer. Note scar is difficult to visualize.
c Post-injection of methylene blue on to the mucosa of the duodenum highlighting scar which does not take up the dye.

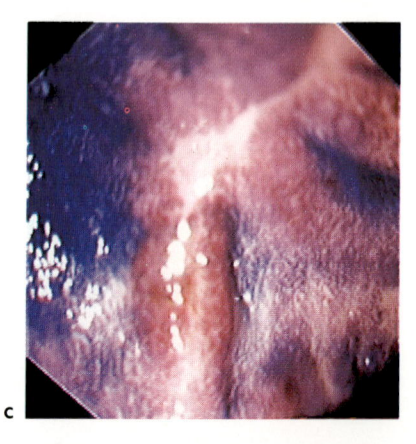

that the development of gallstones, peptic ulcer disease, diverticular disease of the colon, and probably colorectal cancer are related in some way to the western diet, which is rich in animal fat and refined carbohydrate and low in fibre. It has been very difficult to prove that these dietary factors are prevalent in the genesis of these diseases, and the only condition which we know with certainty responds to a high fibre diet is constipation.

The potential for therapeutic techniques

Although the diagnostic and research capabilities of gastro-intestinal endoscopy are very important, it is the therapeutic potential of these techniques which is perhaps the most exciting. A substantial part of this book is devoted to describing and illustrating these therapeutic endoscopic techniques.

In the chapter on oesophageal diseases the techniques of oesophageal dilatation and intubation are described. Before the availability of fibre-optic endoscopy, diagnostic and therapeutic procedures were performed with rigid oesophagoscopes. The procedure required a general anaesthetic. Most patients with benign stricture would spend at least four days in hospital and the morbidity associated with repeated general anaesthetic and repeated dilatation for recurrent benign stricture was substantial. Most dilatations with fibre-optic endoscopes are now performed as day cases, which has resulted in considerable saving in terms of cost to the Health Service. A general anaesthetic is avoided and the risk of perforation of the oesophagus is less than when using a rigid oesophagoscope. Achalasia of the cardia is an uncommon condition in old people, but in this group, at least, balloon dilatation appears likely to replace Heller's cardiomyotomy as the standard form of therapy.

Ageing of the stomach

Morphological change in the mucosa of the stomach is linked to ageing. Chronic atrophic gastritis is much more common in old people than in the young. These changes result in the reduction of the 'secretory volume' and concentration of gastric acid found in elderly subjects. This leads to the displacement proximally of the junction between the body and antrum of the stomach. Thus when endoscoping an older patient the antrum of the stomach appears larger and the body of the stomach smaller than in a younger patient. This does not appear to result in any increased risk of gastric ulceration, but since ulcers form at the site of junc-

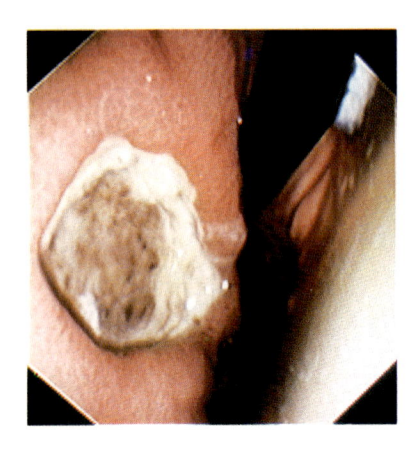

Figure 1.7
Benign, high lesser curve gastric ulcer in an elderly woman. The ulcer lies just below the oesophago-gastric junction and is visualized by the technique of endoscopic retroversion. The endoscope can be seen just above the ulcer as it emerges from the oesophagus.

tional epithelium, gastric ulcers in the elderly tend to be higher up in the stomach. This has implications for surgery should complications develop (Figure 1.7). Both gastric and duodenal ulcers occur fairly commonly in the elderly, despite the demonstrable reduction of gastric acid output with age. It seems likely that the widespread use of aspirin and non-steroidal anti-inflammatory drugs in the elderly contributes to the development of ulcers. The presentation is similar to that in younger patients, as is the management in the absence of complications.

Campylobacter pylori

The H_2 blockers remain the treatment of choice because of their ease of application, rapid relief of symptoms and proven efficacy in healing. However, now that *Campylobacter pylori* has been implicated as a cause of gastritis and the relapse of a duodenal ulcer disease, there has been a stimulation of interest in the use of agents which contain bismuth which both destroys this bacteria and allows healing of ulcers. Whereas in younger patients many physicians will manage exacerbation of ulcer disease with further intermittent courses of treatment with an H_2 blocker, in the elderly patient chronic maintenance therapy is usually initiated. Surgical treatment in peptic ulcer disease is most frequently performed for the complications which occur, for example perforation, pyloric stenosis and life-threatening bleeds.

Upper gastrointestinal haemorrhage

Although peptic ulcer disease is frequently considered a disease of younger people, more than half the patients presenting with acute gastrointestinal haemorrhage are over 60 years of age, and those people dying from gastrointestinal bleeding will usually be elderly. Although it is impossible to prove that accurate diagnosis improves the survival for patients with acute upper gastrointestinal haemorrhage, it would appear likely that accurate endoscopic diagnosis should at least be a guide to appropriate therapy. In an Australian study reported in the British Medical Journal, reduction in the mortality from gastrointestinal haemorrhage by introducing a policy of early diagnosis and planned management, which included information obtained from the endoscopy, was shown to be possible. The improvement was most marked in the bleeding from gastric ulcers. Accurate diagnosis should allow differentiation between high risk lesions (chronic gastric and duodenal ulcers) and low risk lesions (Mallory-Weiss tears and antral erosions). Deciding the need for surgery and the timing of operations is of crucial importance, and techniques which avoid surgery are being explored.

Nutrition

In geriatric practice it is not unusual to encounter patients who are undernourished and who continue to lose weight despite an adequate diet. Some of these patients will be found to have underlying malignant disease, but there is a group of patients in whom weight loss continues despite the absence of a demonstrable disease. It has been noted, for instance, that patients with senile dementia, particularly of the Alzheimer's type, tend to be undernourished, despite apparent adequate calorie intake.

The classical presentation of malabsorption syndromes in younger patients is with diarrhoea or steatorrhoea, but in older patients non-specific presentation with weight loss or generalized weakness and deterioration is just as likely to occur. Our knowledge about the relationship between ageing and gastrointestinal function and structure is slowly increasing and an awareness of the possible causes of malnutrition and malabsorption is important for doctors caring for the elderly.

Liver and bile duct disorders

The conditions causing jaundice in younger and middle-aged people are also encountered in the elderly population. However, the younger patient with jaundice is more likely to have primary hepatic disease, particularly hepatitis, whereas the older patient is more likely to have extrahepatic cholestasis due to carcinoma of the pancreas, or possibly gallstones. The major exception to this generalization is toxic hepatitis due to drugs, the elderly being more likely to experience an adverse drug reaction.

The classical presentation of symptomatic common bile duct stones is with the symptoms and signs of ascending cholangitis. In common with many other disorders in the elderly, bile duct stones may present in a very non-specific manner. There have been several case reports of patients admitted to hospital because of falls, or acute or chronic confusion in whom investigation and subsequent treatment for common bile duct stones has resulted in marked clinical improvement. The cause of confusion or illness is almost certainly due to recurrent bacteraemia, associated with intermittent gallstone impaction leading to transient biliary obstruction. Frequently in these patients there has been a past

Figure 1.8
Number of cancer deaths in the U.K. 1985 from cancer of the G.I. tract.

	Deaths	% of all Cancer Deaths
Colon and rectum	19,520	12%
Stomach	11,220	7%
Pancreas	6,810	4%
Oesophagus	5,230	3%

Figure 1.9
a Mucosal irregularity and bleeding indicative of early carcinoma of the oesophagus.
b Fungating advanced carcinoma of the oesophagus.

episode of jaundice, perhaps labelled as 'hepatitis'. Another clue to diagnosis may be a raised serum alkaline phosphatase or serum transaminase found on routine biochemical screening of blood. The advent of endoscopic sphincterotomy and gallstone removal has allowed the safe management of even very elderly patients with common bile duct stones.

Cancer of the gastrointestinal tract

Figure 1.8 summarizes the total number of deaths in the United Kingdom in 1985 from cancer of the gastrointestinal tract. Cancers of the stomach, pancreas and oesophagus are usually diagnosed at a fairly advanced stage (Figure 1.9a and b) and overall five-year survival for all these conditions is less than 10%. These cancers present late because they rarely cause symptoms until they have reached an advanced stage.

Colonic cancer

Cancer of the colon frequently causes symptoms when still at a potentially curable stage and colonoscopy has improved our ability to recognize lesions earlier. Diverticular disease is very common in older people and tends to involve the sigmoid colon in particular, where it renders much more difficult the recognition of polyps or cancers by routine barium studies. There have been many published reports emphasizing the importance of performing colonoscopy on patients presenting with persistent rectal

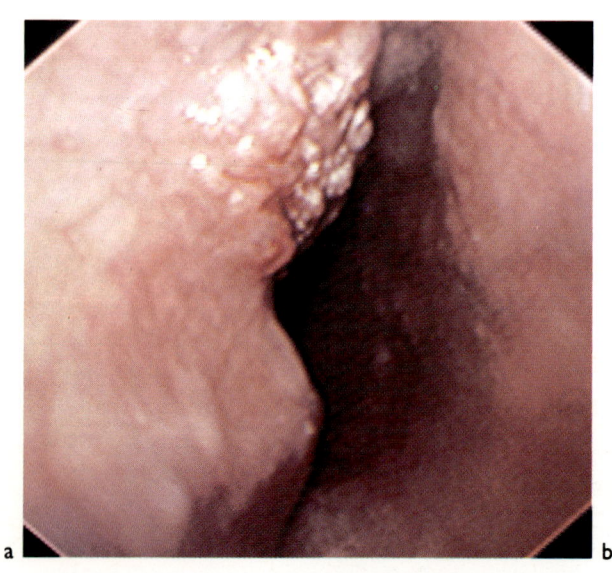

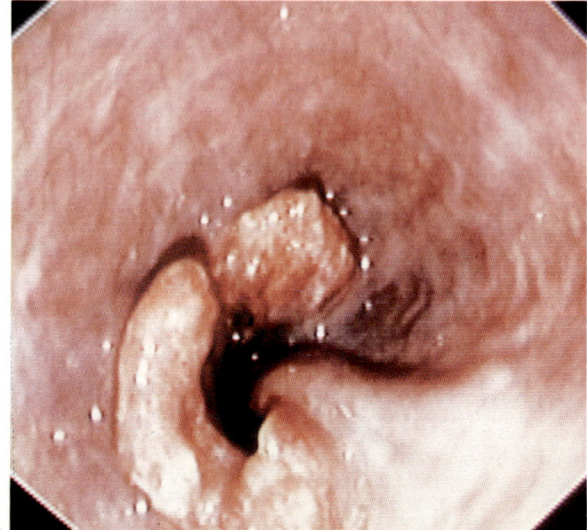

Figure 1.10
a Pedunculated polyp in sigmoid colon (colonic adenoma).
b Diathermy snare placed around the stalk just below the base of the polyp.
c Following application of electro-coagulation, the polyp is removed for histological examination.
d Polyp stalk effectively cauterized.

bleeding in whom the barium enema has shown only diverticular disease.

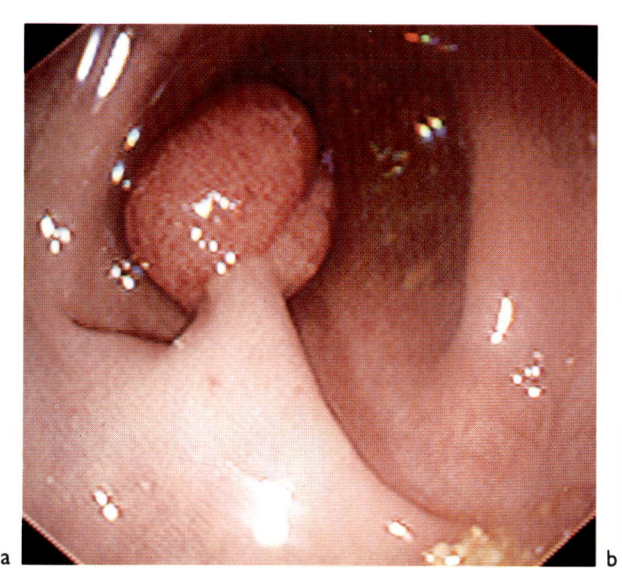

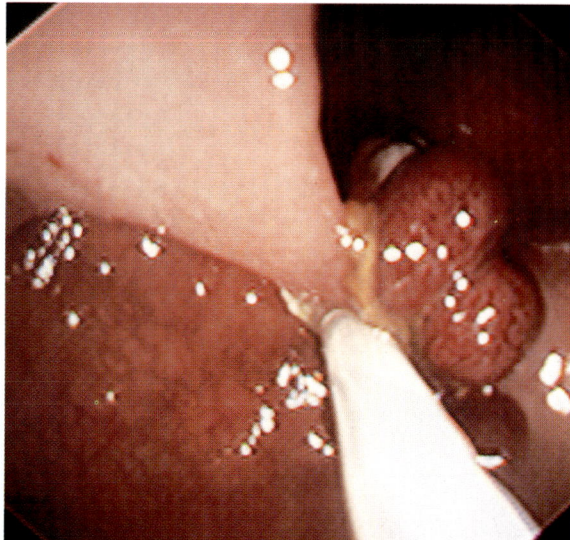

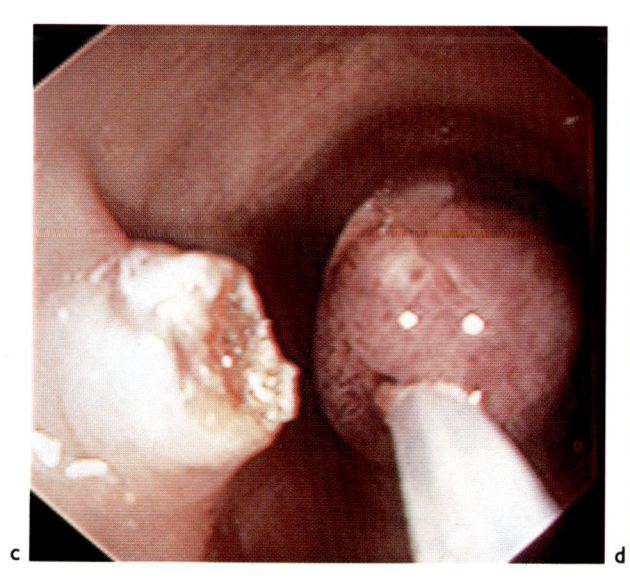

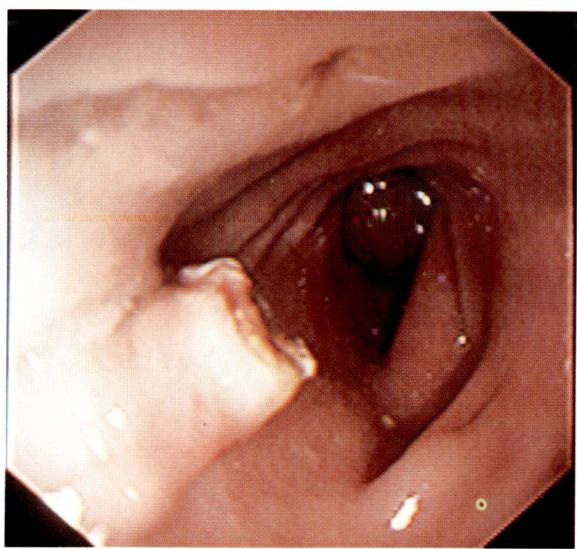

The elderly tolerate colonoscopy well, and good bowel preparation is no more difficult to achieve than in a younger patient. It must be stated, however, that there is a definite morbidity and mortality associated with colonoscopy. The risk of colonic perforation is reported at 0.15% for diagnostic colonoscopy and perforation and bleeding can occur after polypectomy, the complication rate increasing with the size of the polyp. Colonoscopy, therefore, should be regarded as complementary to barium study and not designed to replace it. A great advantage of colonoscopy is that polyps can be removed during the procedure (Figure 1.10).

The overall five-year survival for carcinoma of the colon is around 35%, and for those tumours limited to the wall of the bowel the five-year survival is around 75%. The elderly tolerate surgery well, and it is usually possible to perform bowel resection even when the disease is relatively advanced. The intensive investigation of an elderly patient with rectal bleeding, change in bowel habit, or iron deficiency anaemia is justified.

Faecal incontinence

Faecal incontinence is an extremely distressing problem. It saps the dignity of the sufferer and may be the cause of his rejection by the carers. A recent leading article in the British Medical Journal emphasised the importance of trying to treat faecal incontinence and rejected the idea that it is an inevitable consequence of ageing. Approximately 10% of patients in residential homes for the elderly are regularly incontinent of faeces. In a study from Manchester, eighty-two residents from thirty homes were randomly selected for treatment (fifty-two patients) and thirty allocated to be controls. Those patients with faecal impaction were treated with daily enemas until there was no response and subsequently started on a regime of lactulose and weekly enemas. Those with neurogenic incontinence were treated with codeine phosphate to produce constipation and enemas twice weekly to produce bowel movement at a particular time. After two months two-thirds of the study patients were no longer incontinent compared with only one-third of the controls. Results were even better when full compliance with the treatment regime was obtained. This emphasises an understanding of the mechanisms of faecal incontinence and its treatment is an important aspect of training in medicine and the education of all carers for old people.

Conclusion

Gastrointestinal disease in the elderly is common and merits careful investigation. Such investigations are generally available and many conditions once diagnosed can be successfully treated.

An awareness of gastroenterological disorders and the techniques of their investigation and treatment are important to all medical practitioners. The aim of this book is to provide an illustrated account of current knowledge and expertise in some areas of gastroenterology particularly relevant to the care of the elderly.

Bibliography

Hunt PS, Hansky J, Korman MG. Mortality in patients with haematemesis and melaena: a prospective study. *British Medical Journal*. 1979;**1**:1238–1240.

Irvine RE. Faecal incontinence is not inevitable. *British Medical Journal*. 1986;**292**:1618–1619.

Diseases of the mouth
P L Golding

Figure 2.1
Causes of oral ulceration in the elderly

Trauma
Malignant tumours
Infections
herpes varicella zoster
trigeminal herpes zoster
tertiary syphilis
tuberculosis
candidiasis
acute ulcerative gingivitis
Blood dyscrasias
Inflammatory bowel disease
Iatrogenic ulcers
Mucocutaneous diseases
pemphigus vulgaris, erythema multiforme, pemphigoid, lichen planus, Behçet's syndrome

Soreness or pain in the mouth is a common complaint in elderly people. The symptoms may be due to primary disease within the mouth itself or secondary to another internal disease. The most common causes of the symptoms are faulty nutrition, ill-fitting dentures and drug ingestion. It is therefore important that a patient presenting with oral symptoms and signs is investigated thoroughly with an accurate history including dietary intake and drug ingestion, without forgetting the intake of herbal medicines. A full and detailed examination is also important to exclude other diseases. A wide variety of lesions may be found around the lips, tongue, gums and palate which includes ulcers, bullae, vesicles, papules, mucosal atrophy, hyperkeratosis, gum hypertrophy, pigmentation, telangiectasia, tumours and tumour-like lesions. At this age halitosis is a frequent complaint which can be due to poor oral hygiene, xerostomia or more severe underlying systemic disease.

Oral ulceration

The common causes of oral ulceration are listed in Figure 2.1. Ulceration of the buccal mucosa and tongue is a very common condition. The ulcers may be confined to the oral mucosa or may be found in association with ulcers in the skin and other mucous membranes. The condition may also be found in association with a general systemic disease.

Recurrent aphthous ulceration
This may occur in a minor form around the lips and cheeks, presenting as painful pin-point ulcers which heal in about a week. The major form also occurs on the lips but may also be found

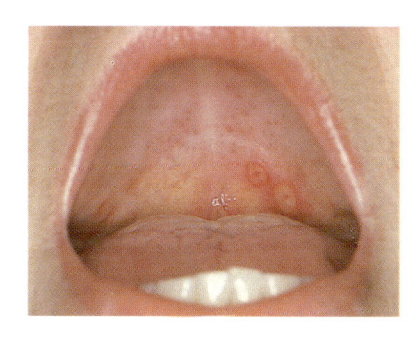

Figure 2.2
Ulcers on the soft palate complicating gold therapy.

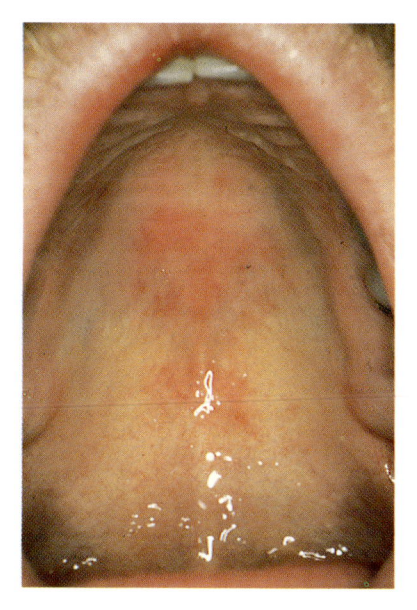

Figure 2.3
Misuse of asthma inhaler causing a sensitivity reaction on hard palate.

on the soft palate and pharynx. These lesions take six or more weeks to heal but eventually do so leaving telltale scars. There is usually associated enlargement of the cervical lymph nodes.

Herpetiform ulcers tend to occur in crops coalescing to form a large ulcer which usually heals spontaneously in about a week to ten days. Recurrent ulceration may, in some cases, be due to Behçet's disease where there will be ulcers in the eyes and around the genitalia. Although normally seen in younger age groups, it may present in later life.

A large percentage of the elderly presenting with oral ulceration will be found to have deficiencies of iron, folic acid or vitamin B_{12}, and appropriate replacement should result in cure. Inflammatory bowel disease should be suspected in any patient complaining of recurrent abdominal pain and diarrhoea who also has recurrent aphthous ulceration.

The treatment of aphthous ulcers consists of correcting any nutritional deficiencies, and the proper application of topical therapy. Chlorhexidine mouthwash, zinc chloride mouthwash and tetracycline mixture should be used several times a day for three or four days. Hydrocortisone pellets are effective, particularly if they are used early in the development of small ulcers. Carmellose sodium or triamcinolone acetonide can be applied to individual ulcers. For those resisting treatment, the more expensive carbenoxolone sodium might be effective. Anaesthetic lozenges, such as benzydamine and benzocaine should be used to relieve pain.

Acute ulcerative gingivitis

This is unusual in the elderly but may be seen particularly where there is immunosuppression. It occurs as a painful ulceration of the interdental gingival papillae and has a characteristic offensive odour as well as local lymphadenopathy. It should be treated with penicillin and metronidazole.

Iatrogenic ulcers

Ulcers in the mouth can occur as part of a systemic reaction to drugs or by local irritation. Those commonly producing mouth ulcers are indomethacin, phenylbutazone and other non-steroidal anti-inflammatory drugs (NSAIDs), potassium chloride, gold, cytotoxic agents, isoprenaline and most drugs known to cause neutropenia (Figures 2.2 and 2.3).

Candidiasis

Acute and chronic candidiasis is a cause of severe ulceration of

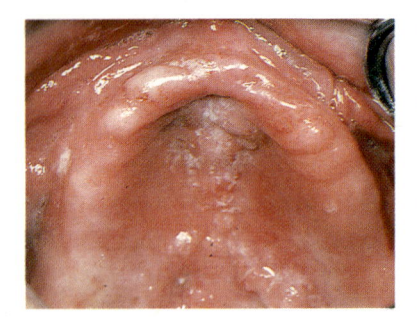

Figure 2.4
Denture stomatitis: chronic *Candida* infection.

the oral mucosa. It is found particularly when there is immunosuppression, in association with severe systemic disease, and as a result of poor oral hygiene, particularly postoperatively. The condition is also common in patients taking antibiotics or corticosteroids. The acute variety presents with milky white patches in the oral mucosa, which on removal, reveal a bleeding ulcerated surface. Chronic atrophic candidiasis occurs as an erythematous, eroded area of oral mucosa, usually found behind the upper denture (Figure 2.4). Candidiasis is treated by the application of topical nystatin either as pastilles or tablets which are allowed to dissolve in the mouth three times a day. In more resistant cases, amphotericin lozenges or miconazole can be used. It is important to remember that in chronic candidiasis denture plates should be immersed overnight in 2% sodium hypochlorite.

Traumatic ulcers
These are characterized by irregular ragged margins and usually heal spontaneously in 14 days. Ill-fitting, worn or damaged dentures or local bite abnormalities are the usual causes, but sometimes they can result from thermal injury or from direct sensitivity to agents used in dental therapy, such as choline salicylate dental paste. Treatment consists of local pain relief.

Carcinoma of the mouth
Squamous cell carcinoma affects the lip and lateral margins of the tongue. It is an indurated lesion causing some limitation of

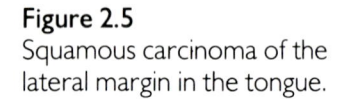

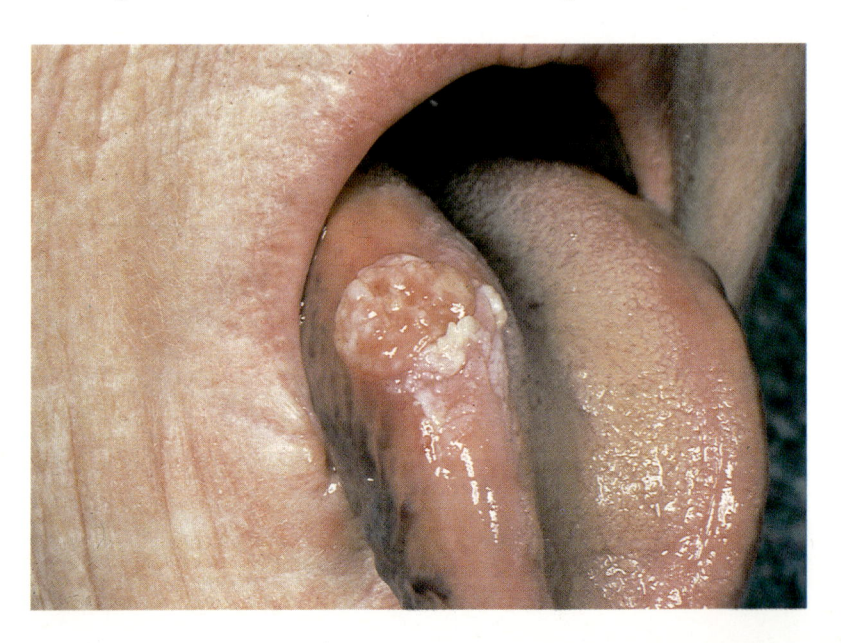

Figure 2.5
Squamous carcinoma of the lateral margin in the tongue.

movement of the diseased area. It is important that if any ulcerative lesion in the mouth does not heal spontaneously after two or three weeks, an underlying carcinoma should be suspected (Figure 2.5). Oral cancer accounts for 2% of malignant tumours but its incidence is declining.

Other infections
Oral ulceration can be caused by tuberculosis and syphilis, which are seen less frequently in the elderly in recent years. In tuberculosis the ulcers are painful, affecting the dorsum of the tongue, and are usually seen in association with pulmonary tuberculosis. Syphilis may present with midline, punched-out, painless ulcers in the tertiary stage.

Oral ulceration in association with other skin lesions

Herpes zoster
Infection with *Herpes zoster* (Figure 2.6) causes unilateral ulceration in the mouth with lesions on the face following the dermatome of the trigeminal nerve involved. Treatment is with local and systemic analgesics together with acyclovir tablets. Although the condition clears, it is frequently complicated by a remaining post-herpetic neuralgia. Elderly people are particularly prone to this condition, which causes concern because it is painful and may last for several years.

Figure 2.6
Herpes zoster involving the tongue and lips.

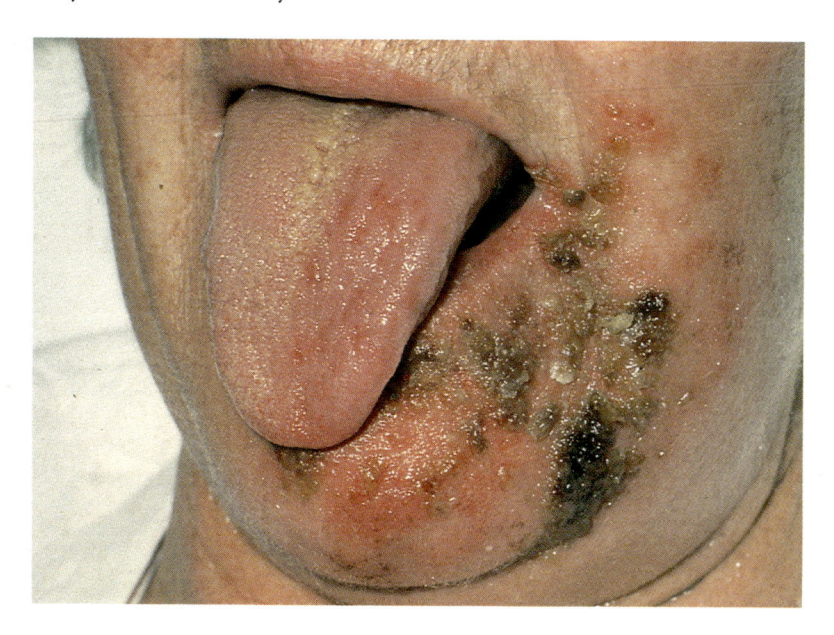

Lichen planus

This may arise in the mouth as an ulcer, as an erythematous patch, or simply as a white area or white striae (Figure 2.7). The oral lesions may be the only manifestation of the disease and may be asymptomatic. However, they can cause marked discomfort, particularly with the erosive variety (Figure 2.8). Typically the lesions are found at the sites of trauma, such as the cheek, and on the dorsum of the tongue. The condition is often drug-induced, the most common agents being beta blockers, NSAIDs, oral diabetic agents, thiazide diuretics and gold. Lichen planus can be treated with betamethasone valerate pellets, or with aerosols applied several times a day. Where there is a severe widespread lichen planus systemic steroids should be used.

Erythema multiforme

This is a characteristic response of the skin and mucous membranes to infective agents (such as *Herpesvirus hominis, Mycoplasma pneumoniae*) and, more commonly, drugs, particularly barbiturates, sulphonamides, antibiotics, carbamazepine and codeine. The oral lesions occur first as blisters and then as erosions on the buccal mucous membrane, gums and tongue. There is often marked swelling and crusting of the lips (Figure 2.9). There may also be severe toxaemia, high fever and inflammation of the

Figure 2.7
The white striae or lichen planus affecting the buccal mucosa.

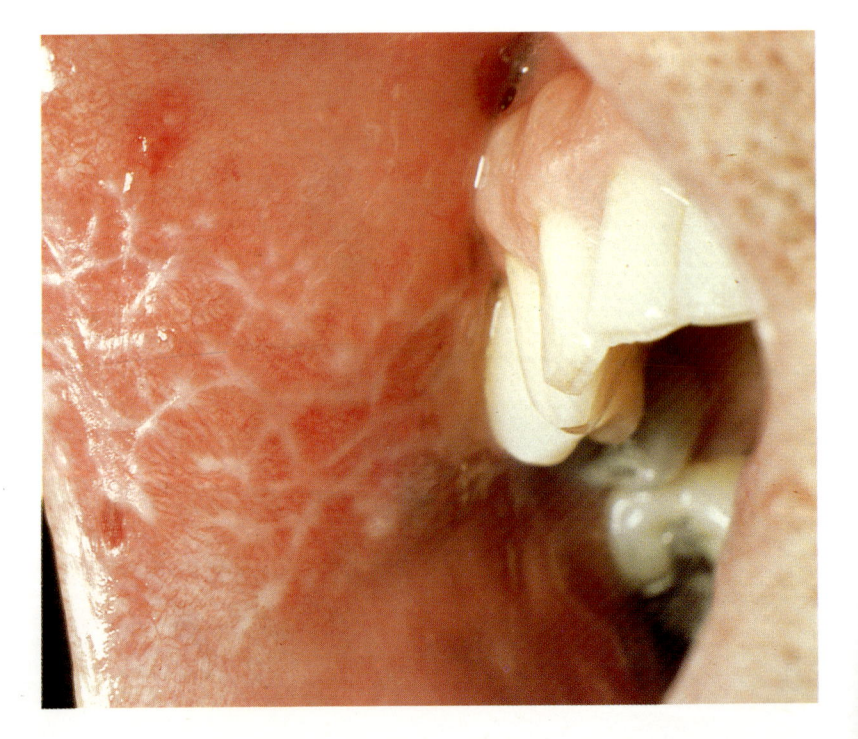

lungs. The skin lesions, initially markedly red, fade and become indurated and bullous. There may be typical target or iris lesions which present as a distinct red area at the periphery surrounding a pale pink zone and a central livid area containing a bulla. Ulceration of the vulva in females and urethral orifice in males, frequently occurs. Treatment is by the use of systemic steroids but there is a significant mortality, especially from a complicating septicaemia.

Pemphigoid

This is found more commonly in elderly women. It produces oral vesicles which rupture to leave ulcers surrounded by tags of epithelium on the palate, the dorsum of the tongue, and the alveolar ridges. It may also affect the oesophagus, pharynx and larynx when hoarseness of the voice and dysphagia result. The lesions may leave painful scars. On the skin the eruption tends to be widespread and presents as large plaques of urticaria. The condition tends to be chronic although spontaneous remission may occur after some months. Treatment is by systemic steroids, usually starting at a dose of 60mg/day and continued until no new lesions appear and a maintenance dose is usually necessary. The dosage required to keep the disease under control varies from person to person.

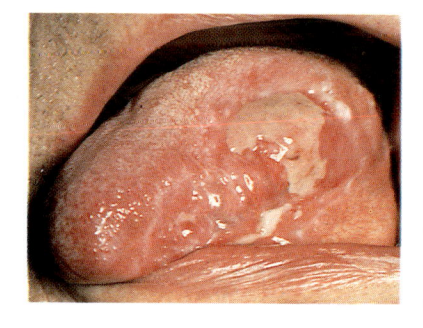

Figure 2.8
Lichen planus with superadded *Candida* infection on the tongue.

Figure 2.9
Bullous erythema multiforme.

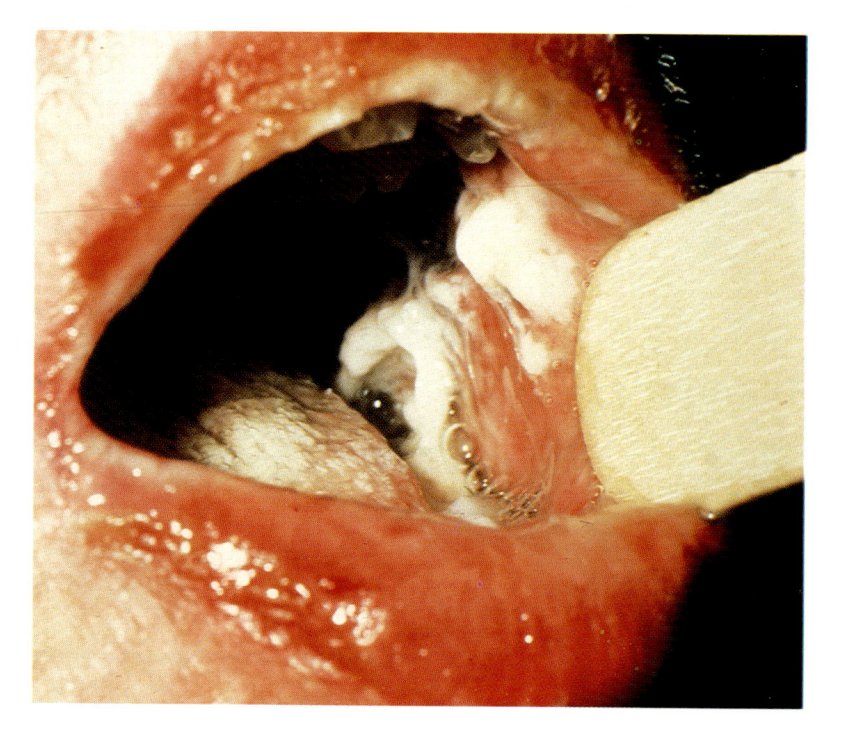

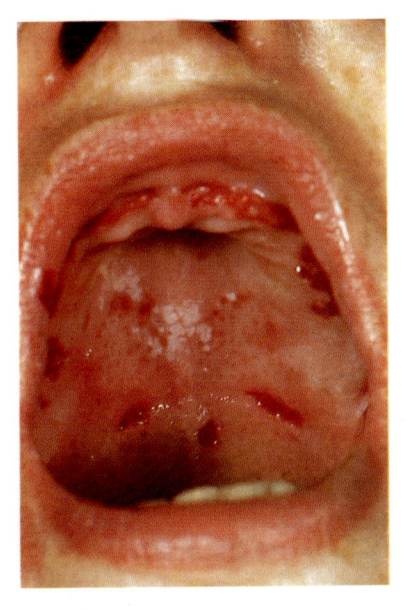

Figure 2.10
Pemphigus showing the burst bullae leaving irregular ulcers.

Pemphigus
Whilst seen more commonly in the 40-60 age group, pemphigus can be seen in the elderly. It occurs in males and females in an equal ratio, and presents as painful erosions in the mouth due to the rupture of thin-roofed intraepidermal blisters (Figure 2.10). It may stay localized to the mouth for months before any other lesions appear on the eyes, nasal mucosa and genitalia and the condition is invariably fatal unless treated. Diagnosis is confirmed on biopsy and immunofluorescent studies, and is treated initially by a high dose of steroids and then a small maintenance dose. These patients are particularly at risk from secondary infection which must be treated promptly.

Behçet's syndrome
This comprises oral ulceration in association with uveitis and genital ulceration. Oral ulcers, usually the first manifestation of the condition, may be shallow or deep and are often painful. The lesions can be single or they can occur in crops affecting the lips, tongue, gingiva, buccal mucosa, pharynx and, occasionally, the larynx (Figure 2.11). The skin lesions may be papular, vesicular, pustular or even as clusters of erythema nodosum. The disease may also give rise to arthritis or arthralgias, recurrent superficial or deep thrombophlebitis, a variety of neurological symptoms and signs, and colitis. Steroids are used to treat exacerbations of the condition but are not universally effective. The clinical course is very variable but mortality is high in those with central nervous system involvement.

Oral ulceration in association with general systemic disease

Haematological disorders
Acute or chronic blood diseases such as leukaemia, agranulocytosis, chronic neutropenia and anaemia may predispose towards oral ulceration. Such ulcers occur more commonly on the non-keratinized mucosal surfaces and are often precipitated by trauma. Some patients may have recurrent ulcers due to a deficiency of vitamin B_{12}, folic acid or iron, even though the haemoglobin value is normal. In leukaemic patients, in particular, mouth ulcers are often secondarily infected with *Candida* and are also a source of septicaemia.

Renal disease and gastrointestinal disease
Ulcerative stomatitis may be seen in renal failure and multiple

aphthous ulcers of the tongue and mucous membranes are often found in inflammatory bowel disease. On occasions there may also be associated swelling of the lips due to lymphocytic granulomatous infiltrations of Crohn's disease. These ulcers respond to treatment of the underlying disease but are liable to recur especially during exacerbation of inflammatory bowel disease.

Wegener's granulomatosis
Rarely, Wegener's granulomatosis may present in the elderly with oral ulceration though usually the lesions are chronic granulomatous gingival swellings. These lesions are all susceptible to secondary infection. The majority of the patients also have upper respiratory tract symptoms – particularly related to the nose, and presenting with nasal discharge, difficulty with breathing, pain over the sinuses, and ulcers in the nasal septum. Response to treatment is poor but some patients do respond to irradiation of local lesions.

Oral ulceration may also be seen in dietary deficiency states, particularly scurvy or ascorbic acid deficiency, causing swollen haemorrhagic gingivae with widespread oral ulceration. Small ulcers can develop in riboflavin deficiency and pellagra. Poisoning with heavy metals such as arsenic, mercury and gold may cause marked pain only in the oral cavity, but small ulcers can also develop.

Figure 2.11
Behçet's syndrome showing ulceration of the lip.

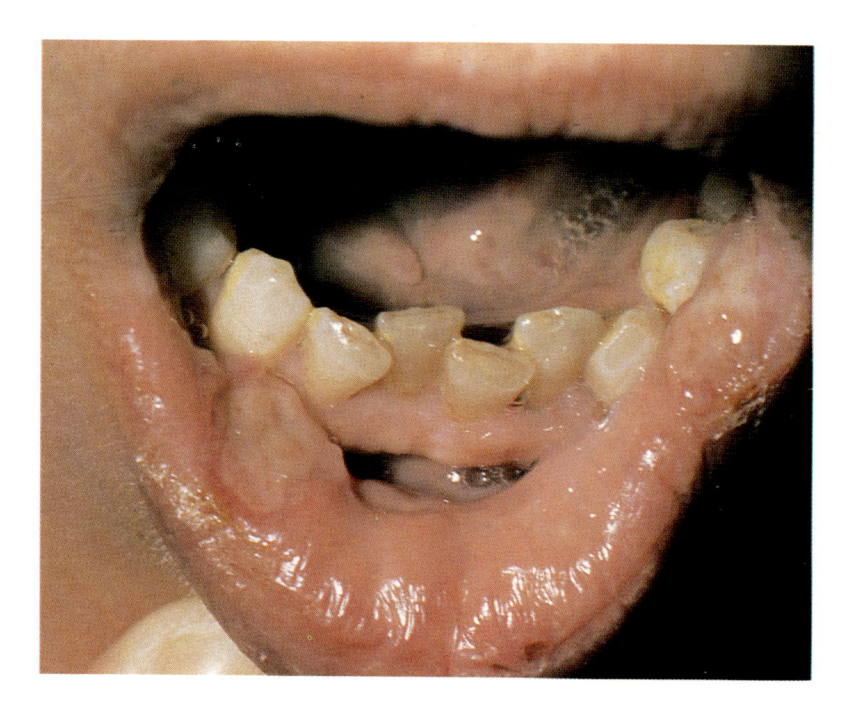

Oral plaque

Leukoplakia

One of the commonest white plaque lesions in the mouth, leukoplakia is found more often in males. Mostly it is seen on the commissure and buccal mucosa, but less frequently it is found on the tongue, hard palate, alveolar ridge and floor of the mouth. It is a precancerous condition and malignant transformation occurs most commonly on lingual lesions. A principal aetiological factor is smoking, but the lesions may also be caused by repeated trauma from sharp teeth or ill-fitting dentures, from the habit of cheek-biting and tongue-biting, and also from chewing tobacco or snuff. It is also found in a higher incidence in alcoholics. Leukoplakia may appear as slightly raised white translucent areas or dense white opaque lesions with associated ulceration. Occasionally, it may be speckled over a larger area with intervening areas of erosion and ulceration. There may be keratosis with minimal inflammation and epithelial hyperplasia. On the other hand, there may be associated areas of dysplasia. Fortunately the dysplastic form is infrequent and accounts for about 12% of cases (Figures 2.12, 2.13 and 2.14). The usual treatment is surgical incision, electrodesiccation or cryosurgery (although this may cause considerable discomfort), or topical or systemic vitamin A. Treatment with 13-cis-retinoic acid may be successful although the latter is associated with some toxicity.

Figure 2.12
Extensive leukoplakia on the tongue and floor of the mouth.

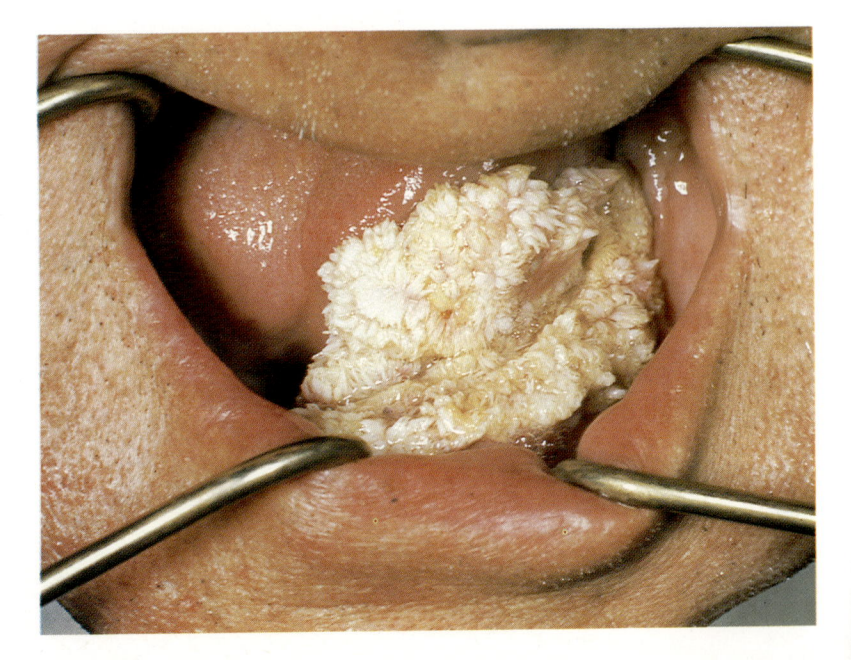

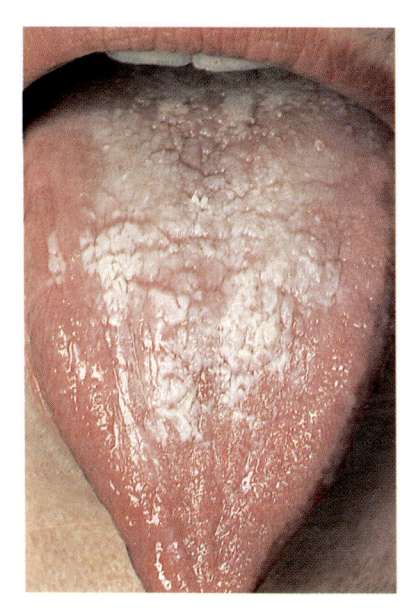

Figure 2.13
Widespread leukoplakia on the dorsum of the tongue.

Figure 2.14
Carcinoma developing in an area of leukoplakia on the lateral margin of the tongue.

Smoker's keratosis
This condition is also known as stomatitis nicotina, or strawberry palate, and is found as a leukoplakia-like lesion on the hard palate of smokers. The palate may have a diffuse white appearance mixed with umbilicated papules with red centres. It usually improves on stopping smoking.

Plaque type lesions
Lichen planus may produce plaque-type lesions on the tongue and posterior buccal mucosa and may be difficult to differentiate from leukoplakia.

Other causes of white plaques
White plaque-like areas can be caused by candidiasis and lupus erythematosus. Sometimes oral papillomas may appear as a white nodule and squamous cell carcinoma may appear initially as a small white plaque-like lesion. It is important therefore that biopsies of all such lesions should be taken at presentation. Similar plaque-like lesions may be found in the mouth in association with cirrhosis. In lupus the plaques gradually disappear during steroid therapy.

Erythroplasia
This may be found particularly in 50–70 age group presenting as a red diffuse area. It is usually level with, or depressed below, the surrounding mucosa. These lesions may prove to be an early carcinoma and certainly many show extreme dysplasia on biopsy.

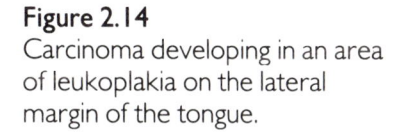

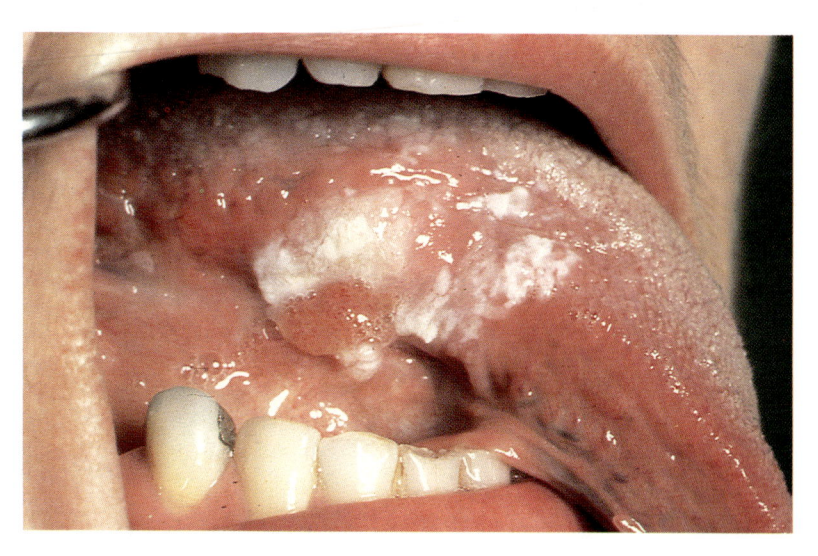

Vesicles and bullae

These lesions can develop in the mouth secondary to infection with *Herpes simplex*, *Herpes zoster* and a Coxsackie virus. They can also be seen in other generalized skin diseases including pemphigoid, pemphigus, erythema multiforme and may be seen in dermatitis herpetiformis where the skin lesions are extensive. This condition may develop in younger age groups from gluten enteropathy, but in the elderly there is often an underlying malignancy. Rarely, primary amyloid may present with haemorrhagic bullae.

Pigmentation

Oral pigmentation may occur as diffuse discoloration or localized pigmented patches. The diffuse form is seen in Addison's disease (Figure 2.15), and is also caused by ACTH-producing tumours. Other pigmentation, particularly of the gingival margins may be caused by heavy metals such as bismuth, mercury and lead. Marked staining of the tongue has been noted in patients taking tripotassium dicitratobismuthate. It may also be caused by other drugs including ACTH, antimalarials and phenothiazines. A localized pigmented area can be due to oral melanoma for which the prognosis is extremely poor.

Figure 2.15
Buccal pigmentation in Addison's disease.

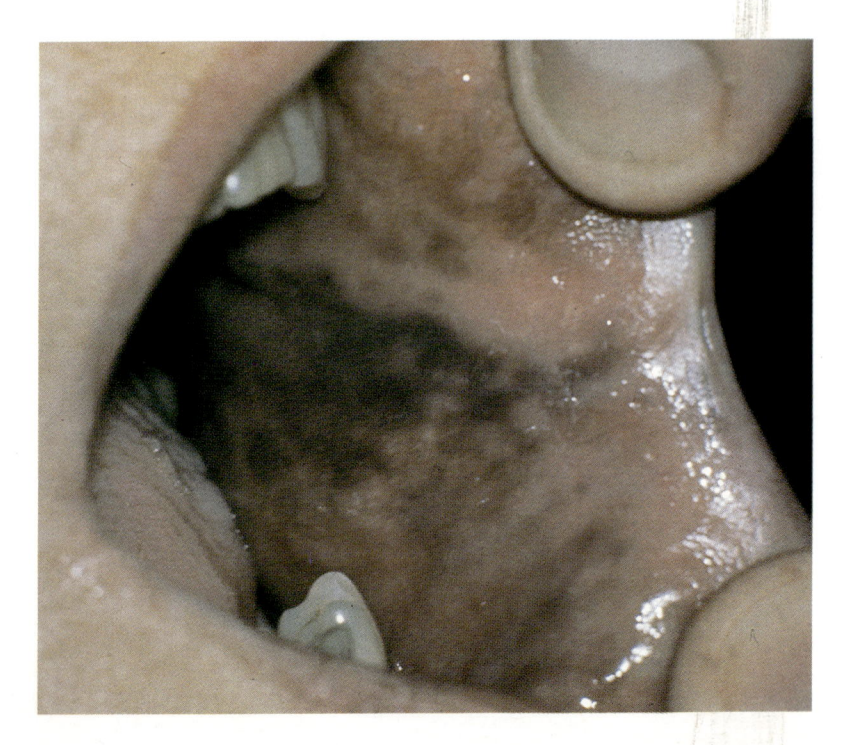

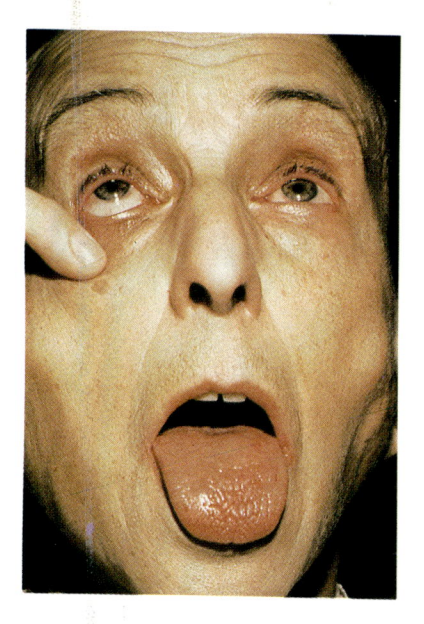

Figure 2.16
The dry eyes and mouth of Sjögren's syndrome (the eyes having been stained with rose bengal) and enlargement of the parotid is also noted.

Xerostomia

Many elderly patients will complain of the symptom of dry mouth, which may or may not be due to true xerostomia. There is often a psychogenic basis for the symptom, whilst in others a dry mouth may be due simply to mouth breathing. In many, the symptom is produced by anticholinergic or antidepressant drugs, but in a few there may be true diminished salivary flow. This is seen following irradiation of the salivary glands or, primarily, in Sjögren's syndrome (Figure 2.16), a disease in which there is lymphocytic infiltration and destruction of the salivary glands. Such patients will also complain of a gritty sensation about the eyes, particularly first thing in the morning, and there may be associated systemic diseases such as arthritis, thyroid disorders and other autoimmune disorders. Diagnosis of Sjögren's syndrome can be confirmed by rose bengal staining of the conjunctiva, by demonstrating a truly deficient salivary flow, and by biopsy of the labial glands which will show the lymphocytic infiltration and the characteristic myoepithelial islands. The treatment is by providing artificial saliva to be used during eating.

This may relieve symptoms when there is a real diminished salivary flow but the symptoms in the psychogenic type are very difficult to relieve.

Sialorrhoea

This does not usually cause much in the way of symptoms unless there are problems with swallowing such as pharyngeal obstruction, or poor neuromuscular co-ordination as in Parkinson's disease, facial palsy and bulbar palsy. The condition can be produced by painful lesions in the mouth, cholinergic drugs and the analgesic, buprenorphine.

Hypertrophy and hyperkeratosis

Gingival hypertrophy is due to hyperplasia or infiltration of the gingiva and can occur in acute leukaemia where it is particularly susceptible to secondary infection (Figure 2.17). The lesion usually improves with treatment of the infective condition as well as the primary leukaemic state. Gingival hypertrophy is also seen in primary amyloid and with the long-term administration of drugs such as phenobarbitone, phenytoin, primidone, cyclosporin and, more recently, in patients on nifedipine. Gingival hypertrophy is usually painless. In the elderly, hyperplasia of the gums is also seen in those wearing dentures where excessive mobility of the plate is present. Bite hyperkeratosis on the cheek is unusual in the older person but where there is tem-

Figure 2.17
Gingival hypertrophy from infiltration in leukaemia complicated by superadded secondary infection.

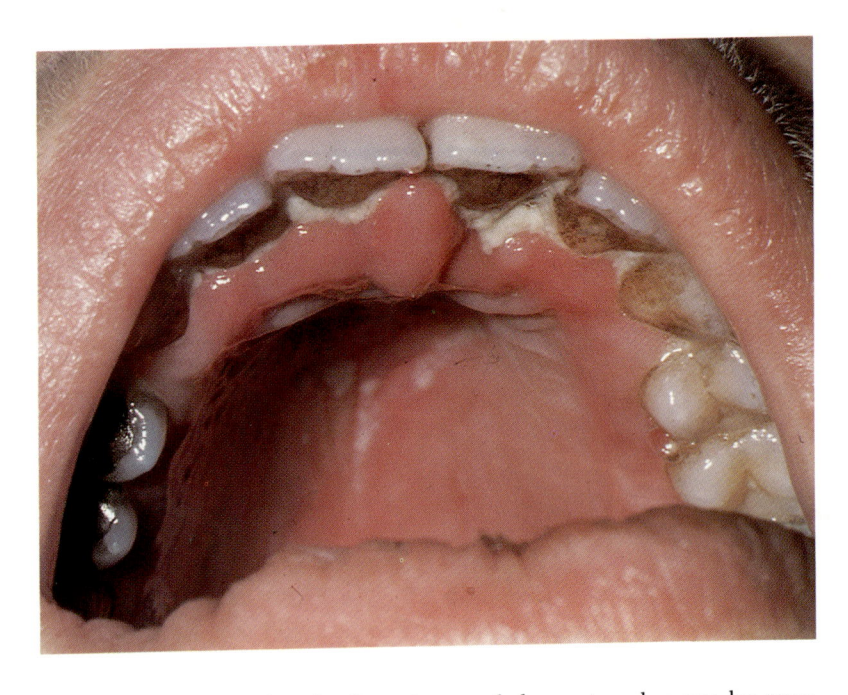

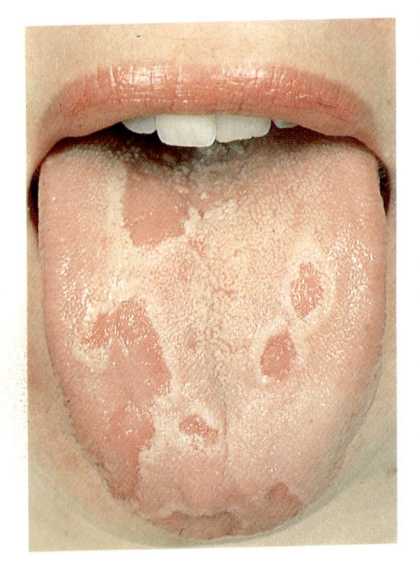

Figure 2.18
Geographic tongue.

poromandibular joint dysfunction such hypertrophy can be seen along the occlusal line of the buccal mucosa.

Halitosis and the disturbance of taste

In the elderly this can be due to poor oral hygiene, starvation, xerostomia, and repeated oral infections. Drugs such as captopril and penicillamine, levodopa, dipyridamole, propranolol, lithium carbonate and certain hypoglycaemic drugs can also be blamed. These disturbances are also found in association with systemic disorders, particularly where there is a chest infection such as in bronchiectasis, lung cancer, oesophageal cancer and gastric cancer, as well as in hepatic or renal failure. Pain in the mouth is often due to local problems but can also be due to trigeminal neuralgia and can occur in many psychological disturbances. It should also be remembered that sensory abnormalities in the mouth together with pain can be due to carcinoma affecting the trigeminal nerve. Of particular importance is compression of the nerves by the presence of Paget's disease in the skull.

Abnormalities of the tongue

A sore tongue with smooth erythematous mucosa (glossitis) may be due to widespread inflammation, anaemia, drug reactions, infection or in association with a skin disease, for example, lichen planus. The geographic tongue (Figure 2.18) may also cause discomfort and soreness due to local areas of desquamation but it may also be symptomless. Sore tongue may occur with a normal mucosa particularly in pernicious or other anaemias. However, in a large percentage of patients with this symptom, the cause is psychological.

Enlargement of the tongue (macroglossia) may cause acute symptoms in angioneurotic oedema or present as a chronic enlargement in hypothyroidism, acromegaly and amyloid infiltration. The black hairy tongue is usually induced by drugs, particularly by antibiotics (Figure 2.19). It can be treated by brushing the tongue with a toothbrush or the application of a solution containing ascorbic acid, sodium bicarbonate and copper sulphate.

Tumours and pseudotumours

A considerable number of tumours or pseudotumours can occur as lumps in the mouth. Hard lumps are commonly due to dental cysts occurring in the jaws but bony hard lumps due to exostoses are frequently found in the midline and hard palate. Soft tissue swellings include pyogenic granulomas and benign connective tissue tumours such as fibroepithelial polyps, fibrous epulis, fibromas, lipomas and papillomas. They may occur anywhere in the mouth being polypoid or sessile but the mandatory biopsy should exclude the presence of malignancy.

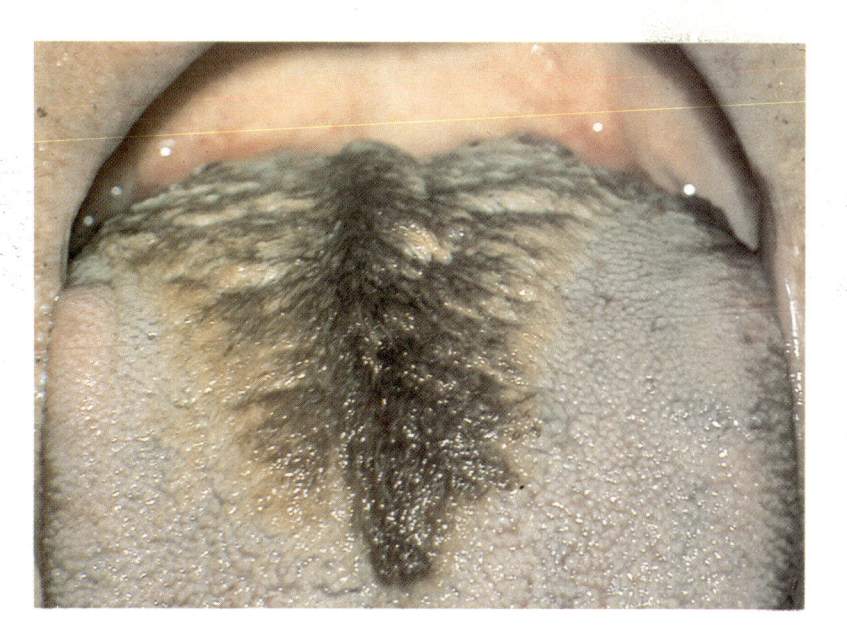

Figure 2.19
The black hairy tongue.

Figure 2.20
Malignant lymphoma of hard palate.

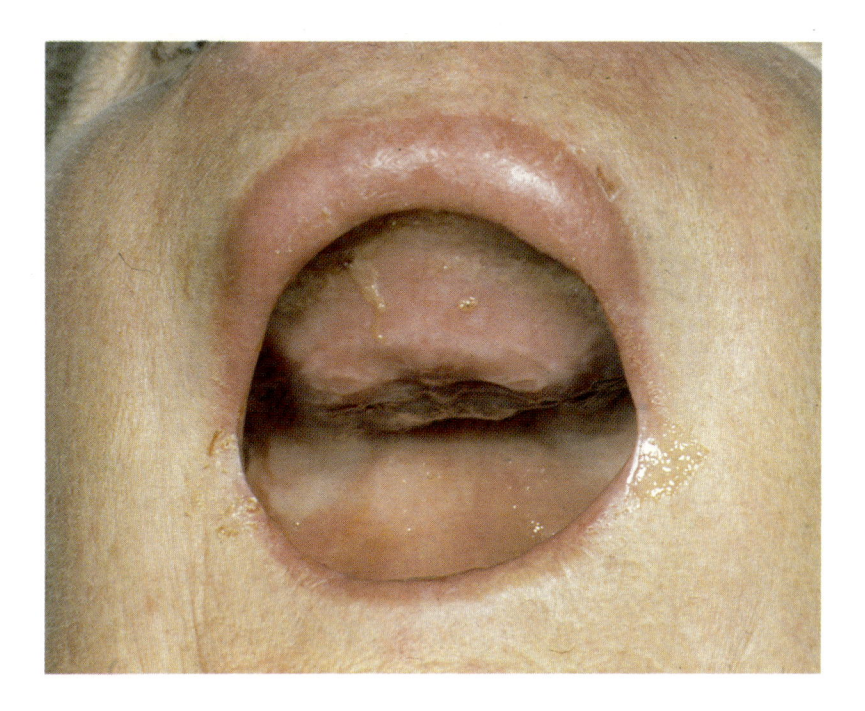

Carcinoma of the oral cavity has a very poor prognosis and is precipitated by factors including chronic irritation, excessive alcohol consumption, smoking, nutritional deficiencies, syphilis and poor oral hygiene. It can appear as a plaque or infiltration, ulceration or nodular projection. Malignant lymphoma may also appear as such a projection (Figure 2.20). Carcinomas of the lip, tongue and floor of the mouth reach their highest incidence in the 70–80 year age group, males being much more commonly affected than females. Unfortunately many such tumours are often well-advanced at the time of presentation. Invariably such cancers present as non-healing ulcers, and pain is usually present but not always. Large tumours of the tongue may reduce mobility and subsequently interfere with speech. Carcinoma of the tip of the tongue is far easier to control than tumours of the buccal margin, whereas dorsal tumours are the most difficult to treat. Metastatic spread depends on the site, with tumours of the oral portion of the tongue having a high risk of lymph node spread, whereas tumours of the floor of the mouth, hard palate and buccal mucosa have low metastatic rates. The management of these lesions is best in a combined clinic involving radiotherapy, oncology and surgery. Treatment often depends on the clinic. Small accessible tumours may be treated quite successfully with local radiation, but surgery is probably preferable for tumours on the anterior tip of the tongue. With larger tumours external radiation is recommended although some centres still prefer extensive resection of palpable lymph nodes. Surgery tends to be used for local relapse.

Conclusion

Oral disease in the elderly often causes distressing symptoms and may be caused by, or lead to malnutrition. In this age group it is important not to miss an underlying malignancy as the cause of the problem, and, in those cases where no obvious signs are present, the symptoms may be due to underlying psychological disturbances.

Bibliography

Shklar G, McCarthy TL. Oral manifestation of systemic disease, *Butterworth*, London, 1976.

Renson CE. (ed.) Oral disease. *Update Books*, 1978.

Scully C. Oral manifestations of disease. *Dental Update*, 1979;**6**:1–9.

Fry L, Cornell M. Dermatology management of common diseases in family practice. *MTP Press Ltd.*, 1985.

Oesophageal disease and the elderly

A S Mee

Although no oesophageal diseases are specific to patients over the age of 65, there are certain differences in the spectrum of disease seen in the elderly which require consideration. These include the effect of drugs on oesophageal function, difficulty in differentiating chest pain of cardiac origin from that due to oesophageal spasm in an age group where both conditions frequently co-exist, and atypical symptoms particularly from motility disturbances.

Oesophageal reflux

Reflux is common and it is probable that as many as 10% of people suffer from symptoms, heartburn in particular, each day. Classically, there is a typical symptom complex of heartburn and retrosternal discomfort on bending or on recumbency. In this situation a clinical diagnosis is not difficult. Nevertheless, a number of less well-recognized symptoms can be present, and a careful clinical history is always necessary to determine whether such symptoms can be attributed to reflux. These include regurgitation of acid or bitter material into the throat, retrosternal discomfort on taking hot or acidic drinks, epigastric pain, and exacerbation of symptoms with certain foods including fatty foods, salads, spicy meals, chocolate or coffee. The combination of epigastric pain aggravated by fat ingestion may erroneously suggest gallbladder disease. A history of smoking or recent weight gain is important. Examination is unhelpful, although it should be noted whether the patient is overweight or wearing corsets.

Investigations
Barium meal. The most appropriate initial investigation for patients with symptoms is a barium meal. This is usually well

Figure 3.1
a Barium meal showing sliding hiatus hernia.
b Line drawing of the above.
c Endoscopic view of sliding hiatus hernia viewed by technique of endoscopic retroversion. The endoscope can be seen emerging from the oesophagus.

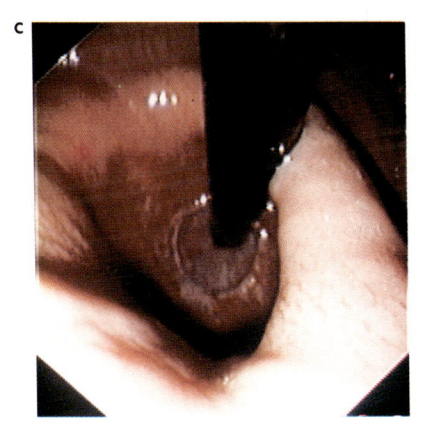

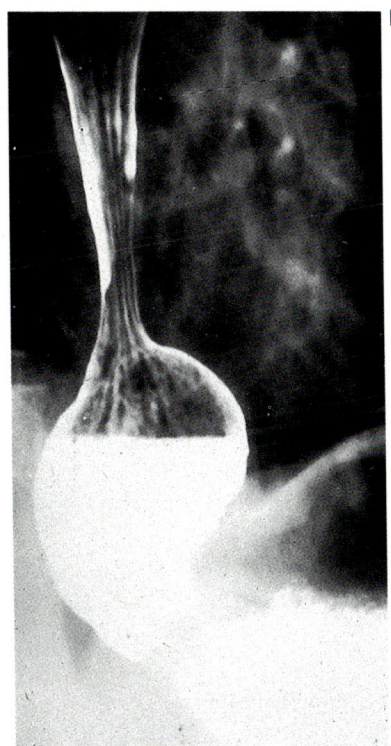

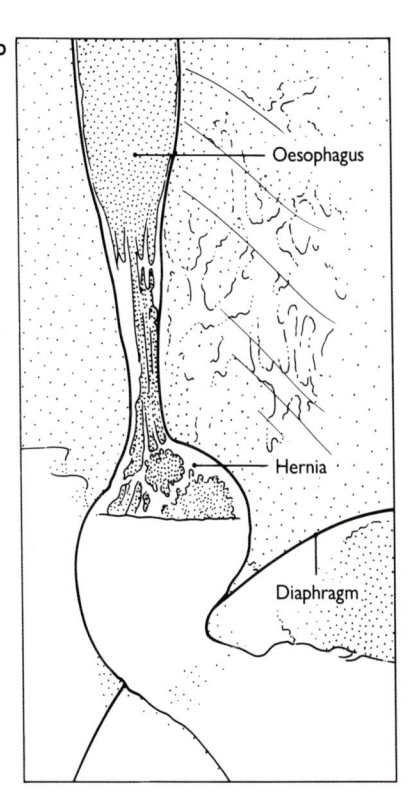

tolerated by the elderly and may show either oesophageal reflux or the presence of a sliding hiatus hernia (Figure 3.1a, b and c). However, it is important to appreciate that reflux and hernia are not synonymous and many patients with reflux will have a normal barium examination which does not in any way preclude the diagnosis. Furthermore, the term hiatus hernia is unhelpful in this context, since many patients will have had a hernia present or induced by the radiologist, and which may have no bearing on symptoms. From the patient's point of view, to be told he or she has a hiatus hernia may be socially acceptable, but it is unhelpful since the patient fails to appreciate the cause of the problem and hence, the rationale of management. Patients with typical symptoms and a barium meal which is either normal or shows only a hiatus hernia, may safely be treated without further investigation.

A para-oesophageal or rolling hiatus hernia (Figure 3.2a) is uncommon and does not lead to oesophageal reflux but to a sensation of fullness and discomfort after meals. If severe there may be symptoms of lower oesophageal obstruction. Such hernias may be complicated by infarction or ulceration of the herniated stomach and for this reason surgical reduction of the hernia

Figure 3.2
a Barium x-ray showing para-oesophageal or rolling hiatus hernia.
b Line drawing of the above.

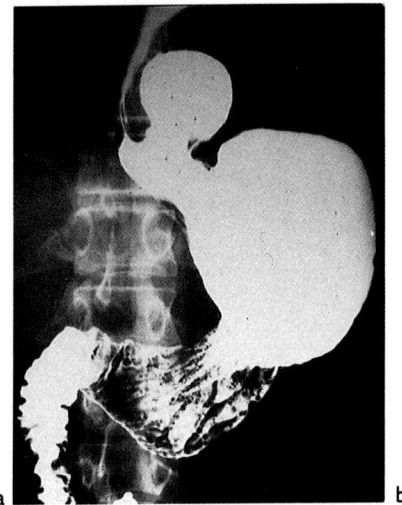

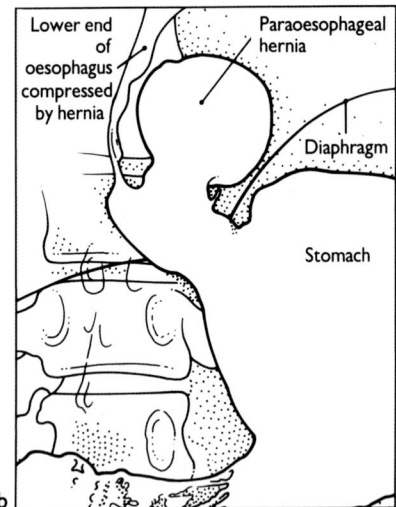

should be performed in suitable patients. Radiologically the gastro-oesophageal junction in such hernias is always below the diaphragm.

Endoscopy. Patients who fail to respond to appropriate measures or have additional features causing concern, such as dysphagia or anaemia, will require endoscopy for further elucidation. As with barium investigations, endoscopy may be entirely normal in the presence of symptomatic oesophageal reflux. Nevertheless, many patients will have macroscopic evidence of oesophagitis which may be of varying severity (Figure 3.3). It is unwise to consider silent iron deficiency anaemia to be due to oesophageal reflux unless there is endoscopic evidence of severe oesophagitis.

Management
The management of oesophageal reflux is relatively straightforward although there are certain important points to bear in mind. The presence of acid reflux leading to an inflamed lower oesophageal mucosa will in turn lead to diminished peristalsis of the lower oesophagus and reduced clearance of acid contents back into the stomach. Hence, whilst the condition may be a long-term problem, a short course of intensive treatment to help to break this vicious circle is useful. The second point is to determine from the patient's history those aspects of his or her life-style for example, smoking, obesity, and the wearing of corsets, for which appropriate advice can be given. (A simple advice sheet which is available is useful in this regard. See Figure 3.4). For patients

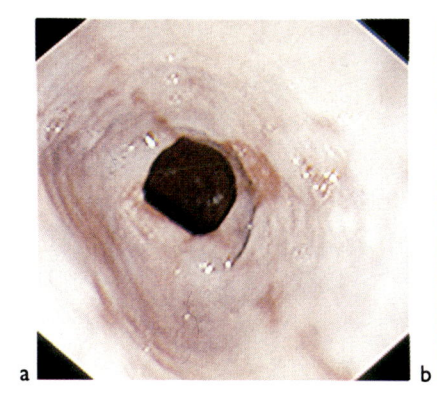

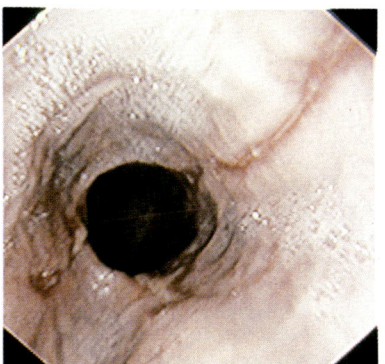

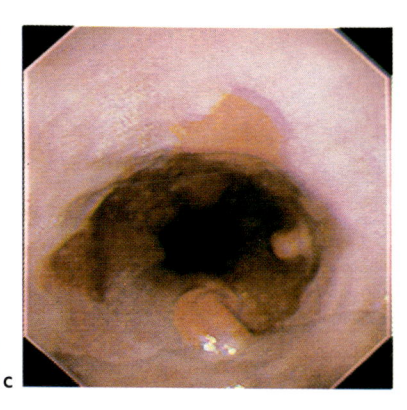

Figure 3.3 a and b
Oesophagitis – two views. Linear ulceration and erythema.
c Hyperplastic polyps in the columnar lined lower oesophagus secondary to chronic reflux.

Figure 3.4
Advice sheet for patients with oesophageal reflux.

with mild symptoms, simple antacids taken as necessary coupled with appropriate advice regarding life-style, will suffice. Patients with more severe symptoms will require more intensive treatment with H_2-blockers or preparations containing alginic acid. Preparations containing carbenoxolone or dopamine antagonists, for example, metoclopramide, should be avoided in the elderly because of the increased risk of fluid retention and extrapyramidal side-effects respectively in this population. Raising the head of the bed by four to six inches during the period of intensive treatment may be helpful, since the problem is exacerbated by a combination of recumbency and lack of nocturnal salivation. Because of the chronic nature of the condition, cost, and the hypothetical risk of carcinogenesis, the long-term use of H_2 block-

DO'S	DONT'S
Stay upright as much as possible.	Avoid stooping, bending or lying down.
Raise the head of the bed by about 4 inches.	But not with pillows which can make things worse.
Eat small frequent meals.	Avoid large or late meals Leave 4 hours between eating and bedtime.
Go on a diet if at all overweight.	
Take your medicine as instructed by the doctor.	Be careful with foods which can increase the amount of reflux such as fat, salad foods, chocolate, coffee, or irritate the gullet lining, for example, spices, alcohol.
	Don't wear tight clothes particularly corsets, long line bras, tight trousers or skirts.
	Do not smoke. Nicotine increases reflux into the gullet.

Figure 3.5
a Barium x-ray showing oesophageal stricture above a sliding hiatus hernia. This proved to be a benign peptic stricture on endoscopy
b Line drawing of the above.

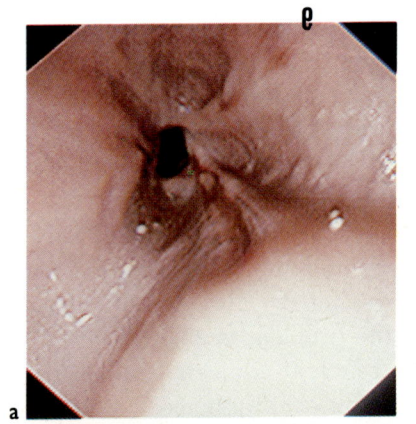

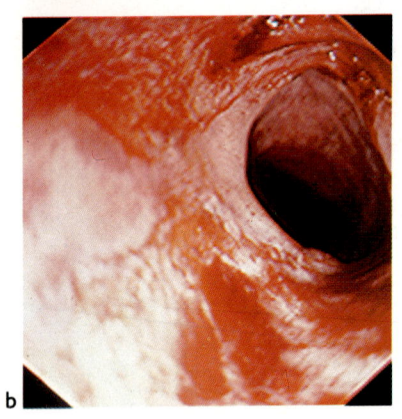

Figure 3.6
a Endoscopic view of a benign oesophageal stricture and proximal oesophagitis.
b Appearance of lower oesophagus after dilatation of the stricture.

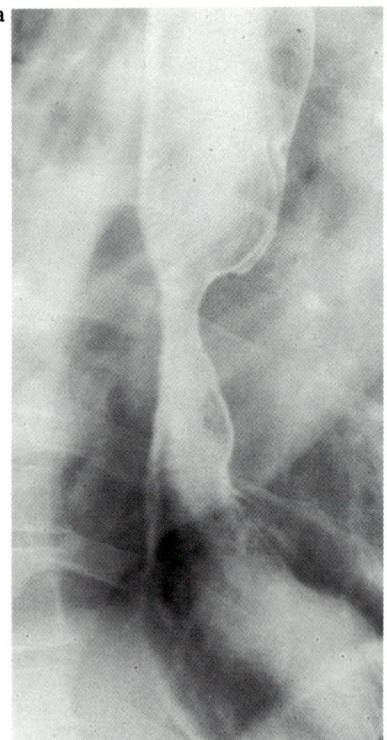

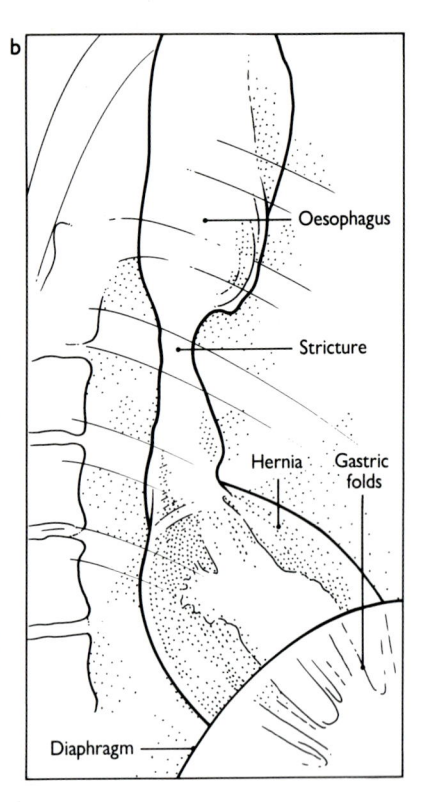

ers is probably best avoided, although for a small proportion of patients with severe reflux, particularly when elderly, the benefits outweigh the disadvantages.

Patients who fail to respond to these measures tend to be young to middle-aged males with manual jobs, for whom antireflux surgery would be reasonable. However, depending on age and fitness, the risks in patients over the age of 65 may outweigh the benefits.

Complications
The two main complications of oesophageal reflux are the development of a peptic stricture and Barrett's oesophagus.

Peptic stricture. This can occur without any prior history of symptomatic reflux. The initial presenting symptom may therefore be dysphagia. The history is frequently unhelpful in differentiating such dysphagia from that due to a carcinoma and appropriate investigations are always necessary, whatever the age of the patient, since peptic strictures are amenable to treatment. The initial investigation for a patient with dysphagia is most appropriately a barium meal. This has the advantage of excluding the possibility of a pharyngeal pouch which may make endoscopy more hazardous, and also delineates the site of the stricture and may give a good idea as to its aetiology (Figure 3.5). Nevertheless, endoscopy is subsequently necessary to visualize the stricture (Figure 3.6a and b), and to allow biopsies and brushing cytology of the lesion to be taken prior to dilating the narrowed segment. This can be done at the same session and is achieved by passing a guide-wire through the endoscope biopsy channel. The endoscope is subsequently withdrawn, leaving the guide-wire in place and the stricture dilated (Figure 3.7a and b). The procedure is carried out under intravenous sedation usually using a combination of pethidine and diazepam. Pethidine is omitted in very frail patients and those with known respiratory problems. Patients of all ages tolerate endoscopic dilatation extremely well and complications after dilatation for benign dis-

Figure 3.7
a A set of oesophageal dilators. A Celestin dilator (upper) and Eder Puestow olives mounted on a wand (lower).
b Celestin dilator being passed over a guide-wire in an elderly patient with a benign oesophageal stricture.

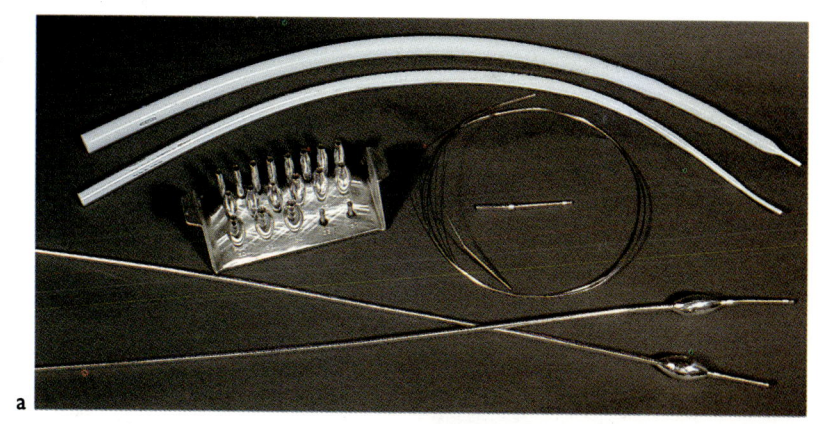

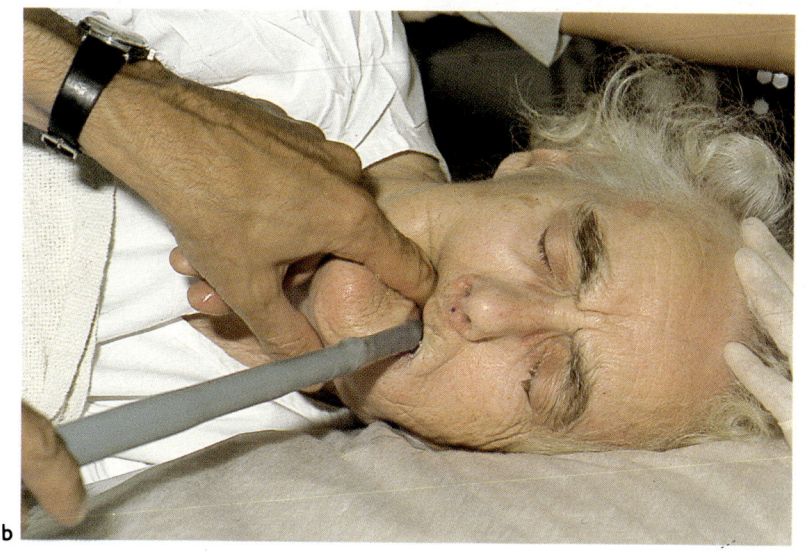

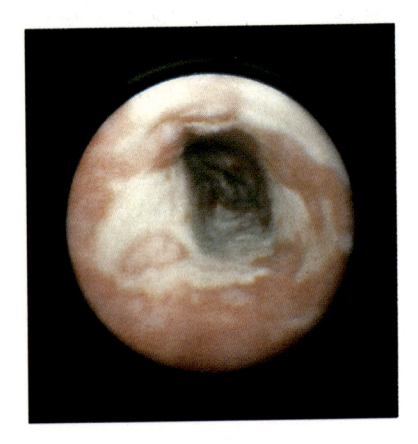

Figure 3.8
Endoscopic view of Barrett's oesophageal mucosa. Note the island of deeper pink columnar epithelium.

Figure 3.9
Barium x-ray showing coarse folds and mucosal irregularity due to oesophageal candidiasis.

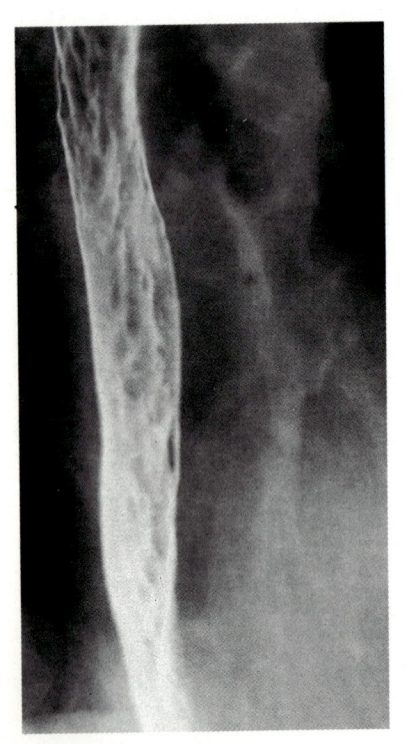

ease are rare. After the initial dilatation patients may require an overnight stay in hospital, although subsequent dilatations for benign strictures can frequently be carried out as day cases.

Patients with symptomatic reflux should continue to receive antireflux medication but despite the presence of oesophagitis and the temptation to use drugs to achieve healing, there is no evidence that any form of antireflux medication minimizes the tendency to form peptic strictures. The rate at which such strictures re-occur is variable, some patients requiring a further dilatation within a month or so, and others being able to eat normally for several years without further problems.

Barrett's oesophagus. This is a further complication of long-standing reflux and denotes the presence of areas of columnar epithelium in the oesophagus instead of the usual stratified squamous epithelium. It may be visualized endoscopically (Figure 3.8). The mere presence of Barrett's oesophagus is of no practical importance although it may be associated with deep oesophageal ulcers and strictures. However, there is a definite risk of the subsequent development of adenocarcinoma of the oesophagus and, as such, it is probably appropriate for younger patients with Barrett's oesophagus to undergo regular check endoscopies with biopsy and brushing cytology to ensure that malignant transformation does not occur, or is picked up early. This is not necessary in the elderly patient since radical oesophageal surgery is not indicated over the age of 70. It is claimed that antireflux surgery can cause regression of Barrett's oesophagus and for younger patients this may be an appropriate option.

Drug-induced oesophagitis

A number of drugs are known to induce oesophagitis and this is more likely in the elderly since there is a correlation between age and increased delay in the clearance of large tablets from the lower oesophagus. Studies have shown that patients should remain standing for at least 90 seconds after taking medication, and that tablets should be swallowed with at least 100 ml of fluid. Oval tablets are more easily swallowed than round ones or capsules, and coated tablets are preferable to uncoated ones. Liquid medication should be considered for bedridden patients and those who have difficulty swallowing. Furthermore, patients with oesophagitis and a peptic stricture are statistically more likely to have been taking non-steroidal anti-inflammatory drugs (NSAIDs) in the months prior to developing symptoms. Other

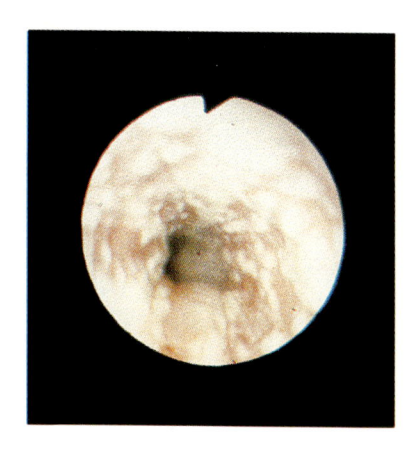

Figure 3.10
Endoscopic appearance of *Candida* of the oesophagus demonstrating inflamed mucosa and patchy white clumps of fungus. (*Courtesy of Dr I Barrison*)

Figure 3.11
A cytological preparation showing candidal hyphae growing outwards from a central fungal ball. (*Courtesy of Dr E Hudson*)

drugs known to give rise to oesophagitis are Slow K, tetracyclines and emepronium bromide. Patients taking these drugs should be particularly advised regarding accompanying fluid and avoidance of recumbency for some minutes after ingestion.

Infective oesophagitis

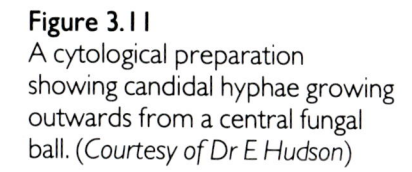

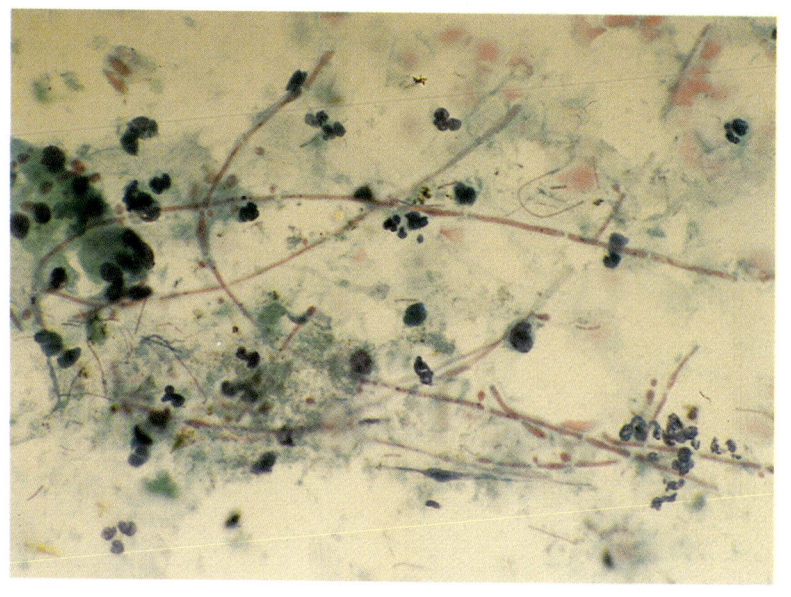

Patients who are generally debilitated or immunocompromised are susceptible to infection by a variety of organisms, most commonly *Candida albicans* and *Herpes simplex* virus. Ten to twenty per cent of patients with leukaemia or other myeloproliferative disorders will be found to have oesophageal candidiasis at post mortem, although this has not necessarily been symptomatic in life. Certain broad-spectrum antibiotics also predispose to the development of *Candida* infection, as does a high tissue glucose level. Frequently, oral candidiasis will be visible and be a clue to the problem. Nevertheless, the frequency of oral thrush accompanying oesophageal candidiasis is variable, ranging from 20–80%. Most symptomatic patients complain of odynophagia with or without dysphagia, and occasionally gastrointestinal haemorrhage. The barium x-ray appearances may be typical (Figure 3.9) although the investigation of choice is endoscopy (Figure 3.10) so that the diagnosis may be confirmed by taking brushings from the oesophageal mucosa. Direct smears will then show the typical mycelial or yeast form of the fungus (Figure 3.11). Treatment with nystatin or amphotericin-B has been used in the past although currently the most appropriate drugs for symptomatic disease are the imidazole derivatives, of which the most well-known is ketoconazole.

Herpes oesophagitis is less common than that due to *Candida*, and when symptomatic presents with odynophagia. Endoscopy will demonstrate herpetic vesicles and biopsies show viral inclusion bodies (Figure 3.12).

Figure 3.12
Oesophageal squamous epithelium showing a multinucleate epithelial cell typical of viral infection. (*Courtesy of Dr AB Price*)

Figure 3.13
a A polypoid squamous carcinoma is seen in the middle third of the oesophagus.
b Line drawing of the above.
c This section from the tumour in Figure 3.13 (a) shows infiltrating squamous carcinoma.

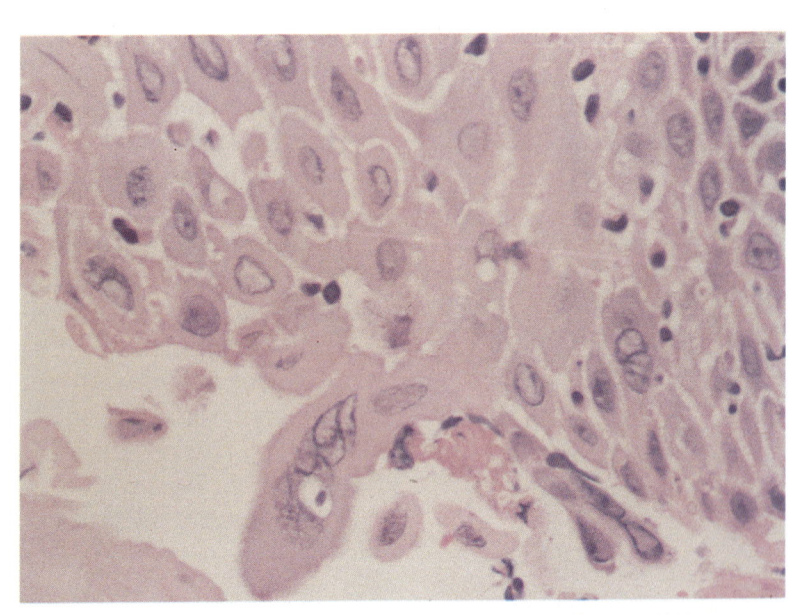

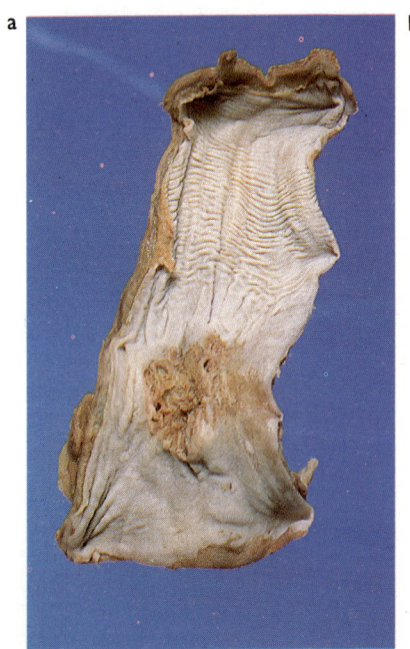

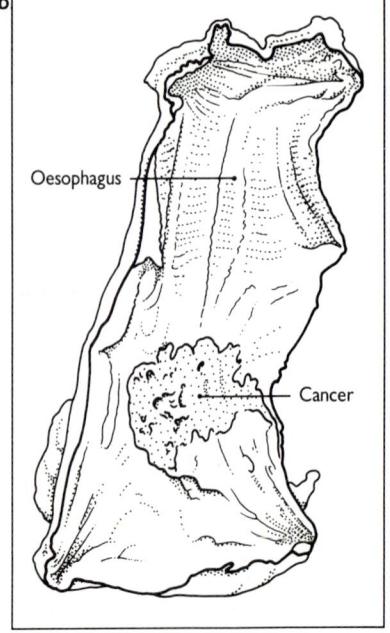

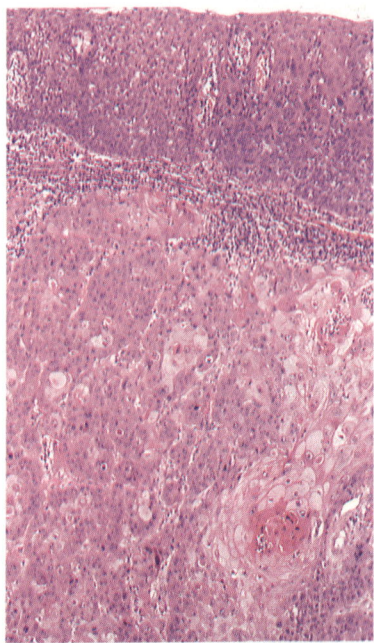

Carcinoma of the oesophagus

About 4000 patients die each year from oesophageal carcinoma in England and Wales, an incidence of approximately 80 per 100,000. Patients are usually over the age of 60 and males are more commonly affected than females. The majority of carcinomas of the upper and mid-oesophagus are squamous carcinomas (Figure 3.13) whilst carcinoma of the lower oesophagus is usually an adenocarcinoma (Figure 3.14). The different histological types have an important bearing on treatment.

Extrinsic compression in particular by a carcinoma of the bronchus can occur but considering the high incidence of the condition, it rarely results in dysphagia.

Figure 3.14
a An adenocarcinoma at the cardio-oesophageal junction.
b Line drawing of the above.
c Histology shows intact non-malignant squamous oesophageal epithelium at the top of the picture with infiltrating adenocarcinoma beneath it.

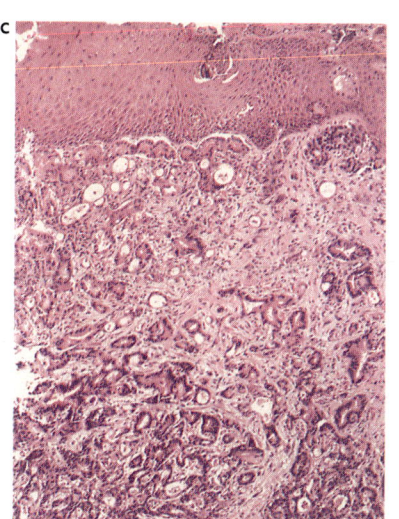

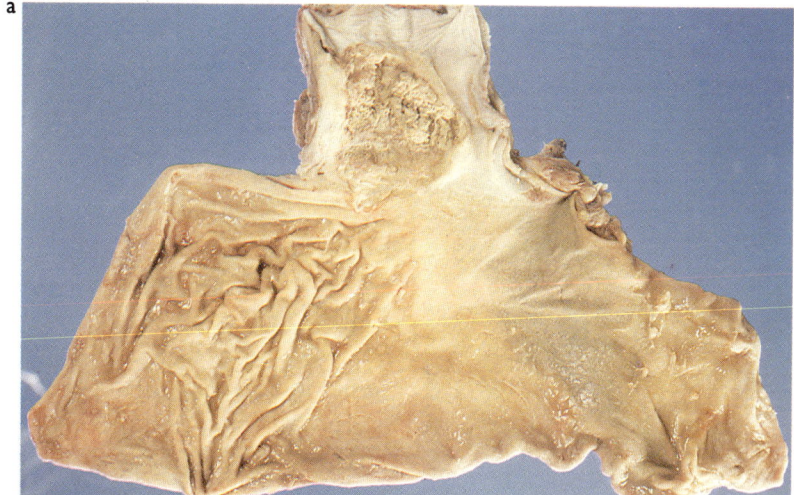

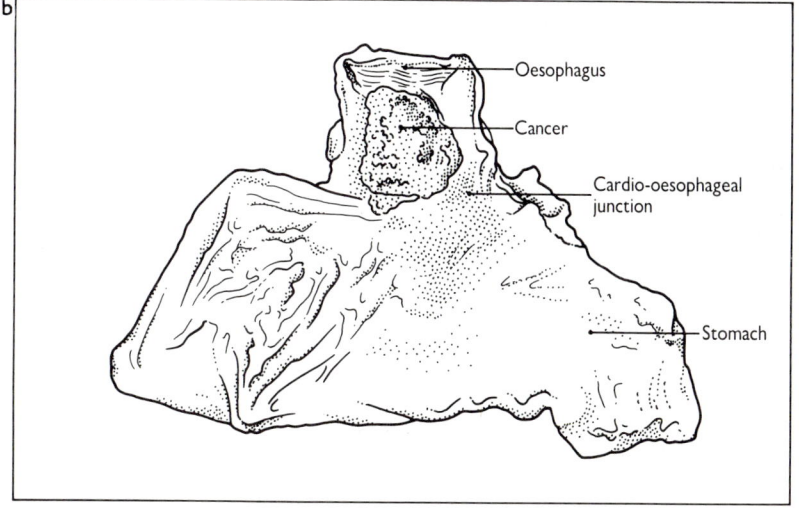

Figure 3.15
a Barium swallow showing stricture of the lower oesophagus due to adenocarcinoma.
b Line drawing of the above.

Figure 3.16
Barium swallow showing large protuberant and polypoid neoplasm occluding the lower oesophagus (arrowed).

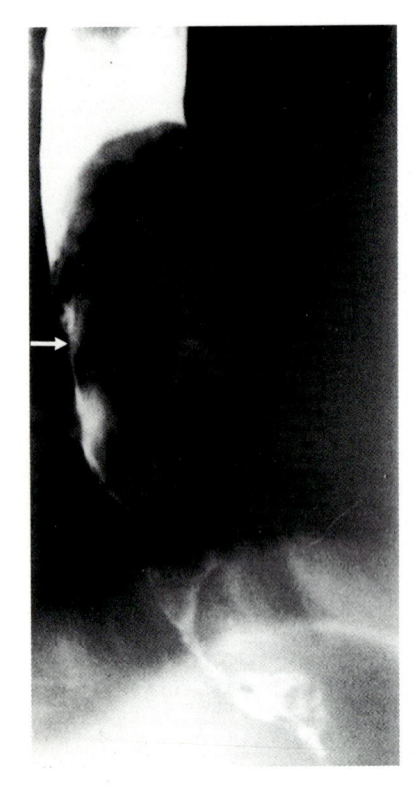

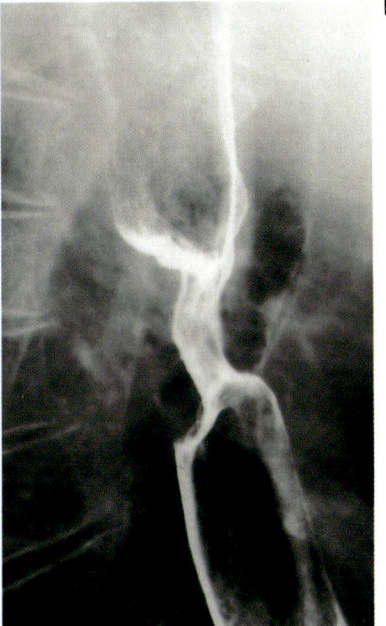

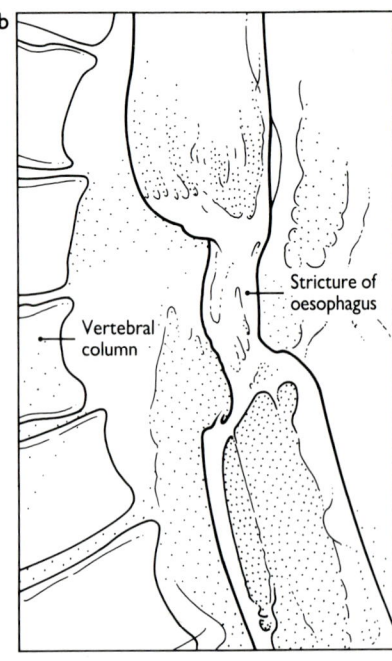

It is probable that most lower oesophageal carcinomas arise from the stomach, although true adenocarcinoma of the oesophagus does exist, for example, arising from Barrett's mucosa. Eighty per cent of patients will present with dysphagia, although 20% will never have had any difficulty with swallowing. Half the patients may experience pain in the chest or upper abdomen, and, rarely, regurgitation is a problem. Most patients will have lost a significant amount of weight at the time of presentation and may well have had symptoms for up to six months. The radiological appearances of an oesophageal carcinoma are varied, ranging from narrowed strictures (Figure 3.15) to poly-

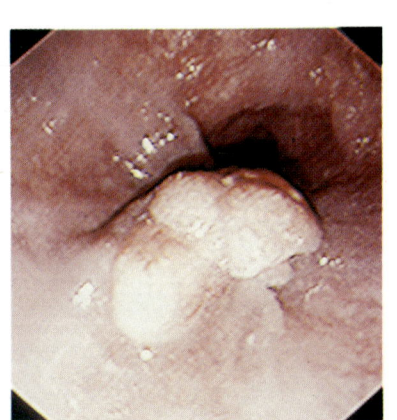

Figure 3.17
Endoscopic view of squamous carcinoma of the oesophagus showing irregular friable neoplastic tissue.

Figure 3.18
Oesophageal endoprosthesis mounted on a wand prior to insertion over guide-wire. Note distal flange and proximal funnel (arrowed) to prevent upward or downward displacement of prosthesis when *in situ*.

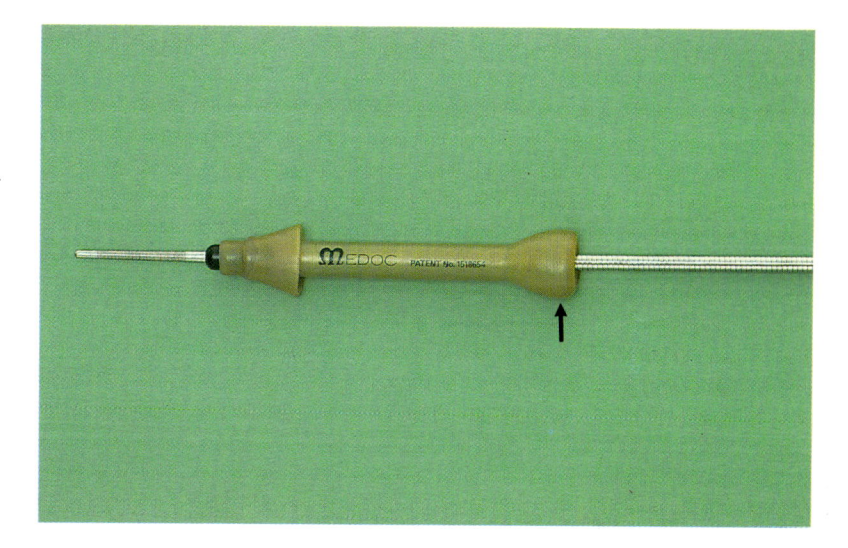

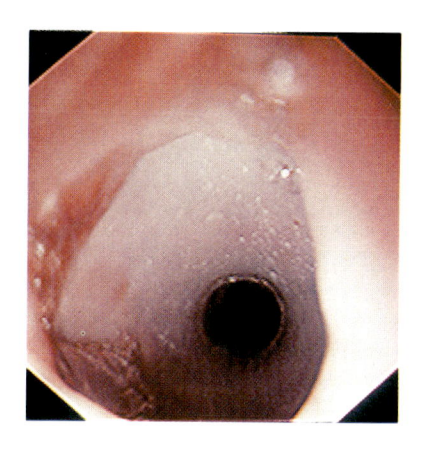

Figure 3.19
Endoscopic view of prosthesis in place above tumour. The upper flange of the prosthesis is clearly visible.

poid protuberances within the oesophageal lumen (Figure 3.16). Endoscopy with brushing cytology and biopsy is always necessary to confirm the radiological findings, and to determine the exact histological type of tumour present (Figure 3.17). Whilst individually brushing cytology is probably more accurate than biopsy, the best approach is to use a combination of both. The management of oesophageal carcinomas is difficult since, if curative resection is attempted, the mortality in patients over the age of 70 becomes prohibitive. Even palliative surgery, although giving good symptomatic results, has a very high operative morbidity and mortality. The majority of tumours will have lymph node spread at the time of diagnosis, and it has been calculated from a large review of the literature that of 100 patients with an oesophageal carcinoma, 58% will be explored, 39% resected and only 26% leave hospital with the tumour excised. Meanwhile, 18% will survive for one year, 9% for two years and only 4% have a five-year survival. Patients who by virtue of age or general debility are deemed a poor operative risk are likely to have a far worse outcome than this.

For patients with a squamous carcinoma of the oesophagus, management is facilitated by the fact that these tumours are radiosensitive and elderly patients should therefore be referred direct for radiotherapy, since five-year survival from this form of treatment is comparable to that of surgery.

Patients with an obstructing adenocarcinoma, even if not suitable for resection, require palliative treatment. This is most easily accomplished in the elderly and infirm by means of either the insertion of a prosthesis endoscopically (Figures 3.18 and 3.19) or, if the tumour is protuberant and facilities available, by laser obliteration (Figures 3.20a to d). Both these procedures can be carried out endoscopically under intravenous sedation, and the risks are therefore far less than for palliative intubation performed under general anaesthetic or at open operation. The complications of tube insertion include oesophageal perforation at the time of the procedure. This is not necessarily catastrophic since if the tube can be placed it will act as a stent across the perforation allowing it to heal in a proportion of patients. Longer term com-

Figure 3.20
a Proliferative carcinoma of the lower (arrowed) oesophagus prior to laser therapy. (*Courtesy of Dr S Bown*)
b Barium swallow, same patient, now showing a substantial oesophageal lumen after laser destruction of tumour (*Courtesy of Dr S Bown*)
c Endoscopic view of adenocarcinoma of oesophagus causing complete obstruction of the oesophagus.
d Adenocarcinoma of the lower oesophagus after YAG laser obliteration of tumour. An oesophageal lumen is now visible.

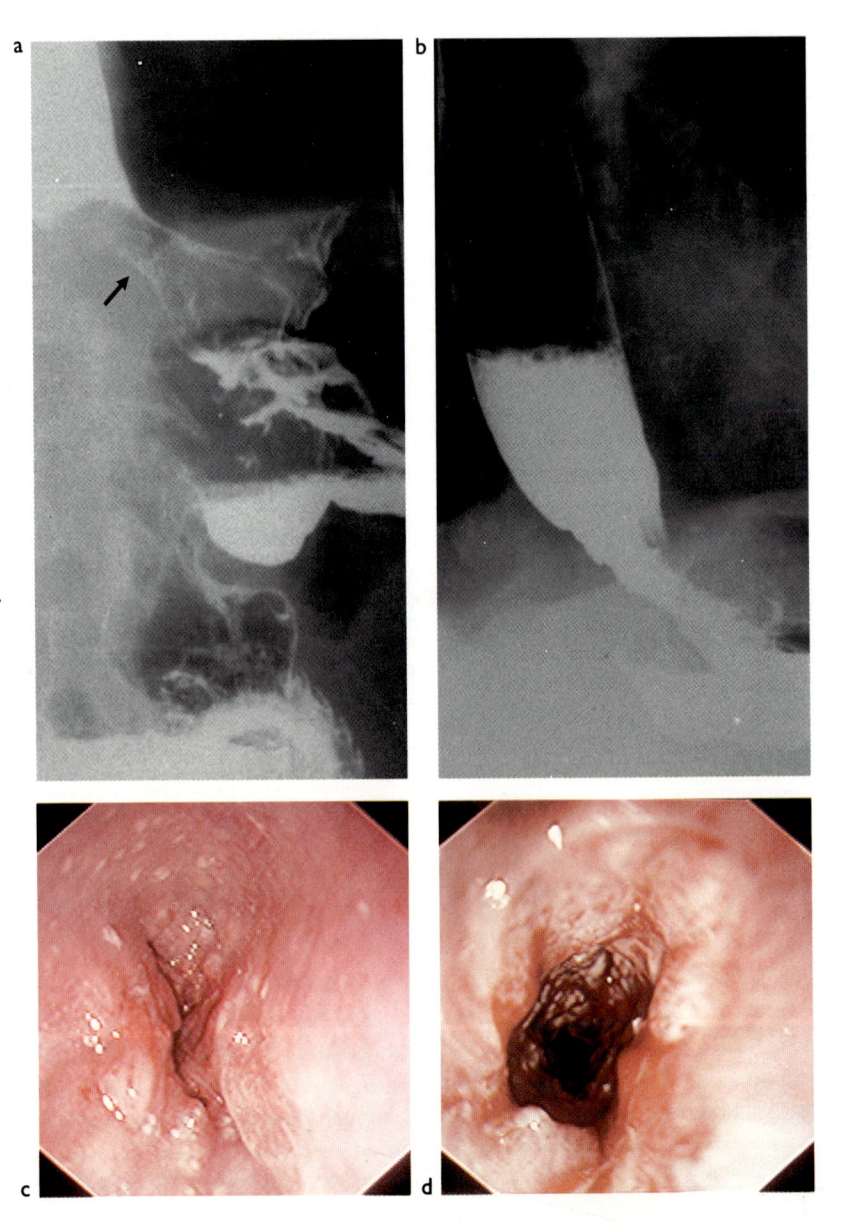

plications include tube blockage with impacted food, migration of the tube through the gastrointestinal tract and erosion through into the mediastinum. Other than food impaction these complications are rare. Patients with a tube should be advised to wash their food down with frequent, preferably fizzy, drinks. They should chew their food well and avoid large boluses of meat or bread. Adequate dentition is vital. A proportion of patients do well with repeated endoscopic dilatation alone.

Using such techniques no patients should die unable to swallow their own saliva.

Motility disorders of the oesophagus

Oropharyngeal dysphagia
Motility disorders of the pharyngo-oesophageal region are not uncommon in the elderly. Disturbed motility can lead to tracheal aspiration or nasal regurgitation of boluses, particularly liquids. Subsequent fear of the consequences of this can lead to inadequate nutrition and recurrent respiratory infections. A number of conditions lead to oropharyngeal dysphagia including cerebrovascular accidents, polymyositis, Parkinson's disease, myasthe-

Figure 3.21
a Barium swallow showing lateral and anterioposterior view of the pharyngeal pouch.
b Line drawing of the above.

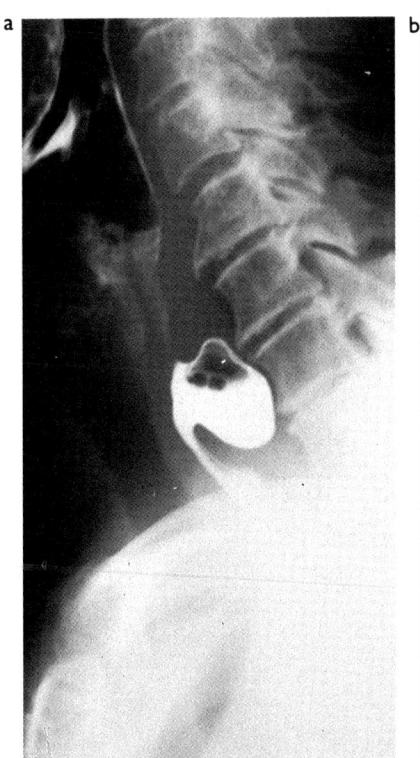

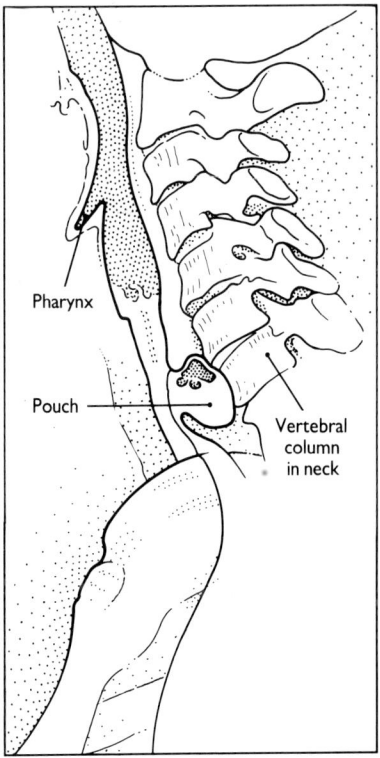

nia gravis and hypothyroidism. Nevertheless there remains a group of individuals in whom associated conditions have been eliminated who continue to have difficulty swallowing, involving the pharynx and upper oesophageal sphincter. This has been termed cricopharyngeal achalasia. Investigation by manometry of the upper oesophageal sphincter is difficult although there is no doubt that the upper oesophageal sphincter pressure falls markedly with age rendering the sphincter more hypotonic. Management of such patients is extremely difficult although a proportion of patients with oropharyngeal dysphagia will benefit from a cricopharyngeal myotomy if they are considered to be a good anaesthetic risk.

Pharyngeal pouch (Zenker's diverticulum)

Hypopharyngeal diverticula occur predominantly in elderly patients, the average age being 74. It is thought that a combination of a weak point in the pharyngeal wall and motility disorders of the pharyngo-oesophageal region in the elderly are amongst the factors involved in the pathogenesis of these pouches, although

Figure 3.22
Diagramatic representation of oesophageal manometry tracing in achalasia. Note the non-sequential contractions of oesophagus body and increased resting lower oesophageal pressure

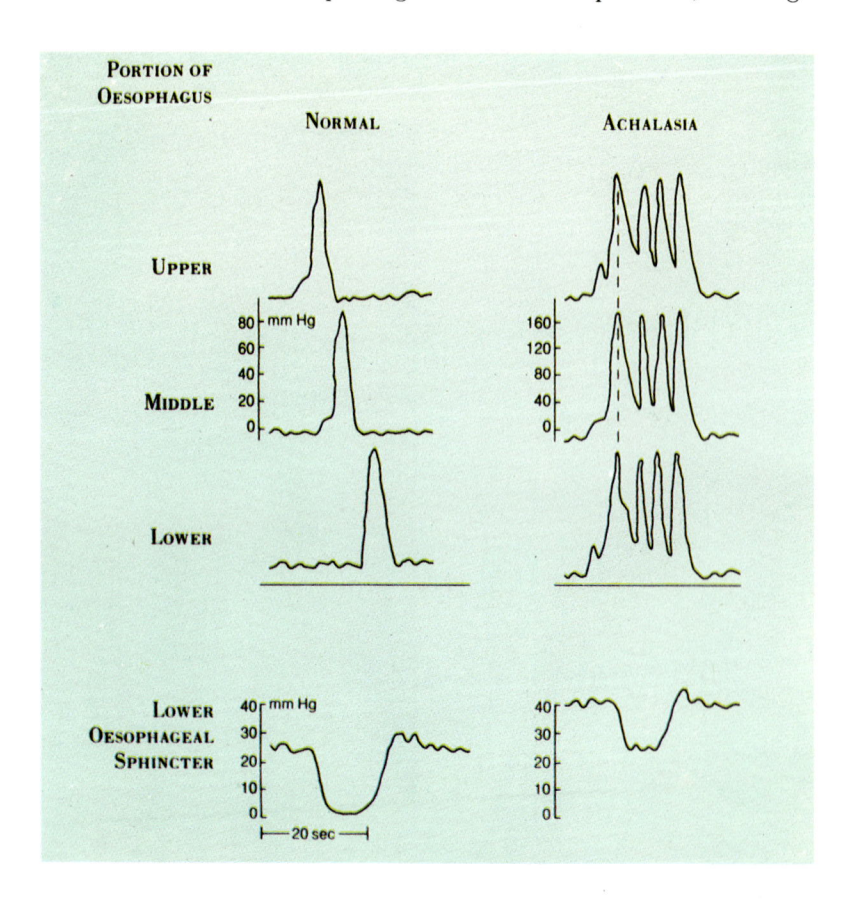

the exact aetiology remains unknown. They tend to occur more commonly on the left side of the neck, and there is a suggestion that they are related to a patient's handedness. Patients present with dysphagia or they may notice a gurgling in the neck on swallowing. If the pouch is large enough it may be palpable. A barium x-ray is the most important investigation, and should be carried out in preference to endoscopy in order to avoid blind perforation of the diverticulum (Figure 3.21). If the patient is fit enough then treatment is surgical with excision of the pouch, which may or may not be combined with a cricopharyngeal myotomy.

Achalasia of the cardia

The aetiology of this uncommon condition remains unknown. It is manifested by three abnormalities of oesophageal function: aperistalsis, partial or incomplete relaxation of the lower oesophageal sphincter, and an increased resting lower oesophageal sphincter pressure (Figure 3.22). Although the condition frequently occurs in young patients, no age is exempt and in the elderly exclusion of a carcinoma of the cardia mimicking achalasia is imperative. Patients usually present with progressive dysphagia, which is frequently the same for both solids and liquids, as distinct from dysphagia due to a carcinoma. This may be accompanied by chest pain, although this is more frequent in younger people. Nocturnal cough due to aspiration of retained oesophageal contents is common, and can lead to recurrent aspiration pneumonia. This in turn may be a presenting feature. A plain chest x-ray may be a clue to the diagnosis for, as well as showing evidence of consolidation, there may also be a mediastinal shadow with fluid level present, and an absent gastric air bubble is characteristic (Figure 3.23a and b).

Figure 3.23
a Plain chest x-ray (postero-anterior).
b Lateral chest x-ray showing widened mediastinum and fluid level due to dilated oesophagus containing residue of food and fluid.

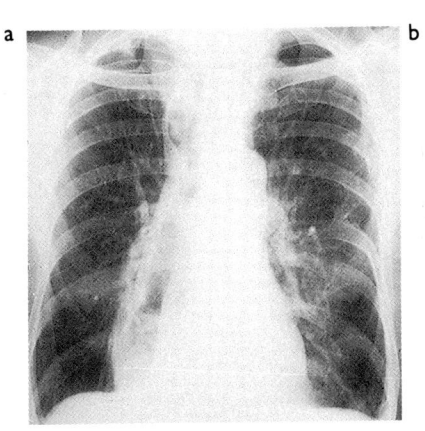

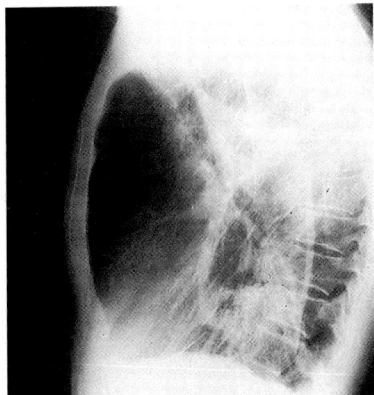

Investigations. For practical purposes the most important investigation is a barium x-ray (Figure 3.24), followed by a careful endoscopy paying particular attention to the oesophago-gastric junction. Retroflexion of the endoscope within the stomach to look at this region from below is important, as small carcinomas at this site can result in the radiological appearances of achalasia. Oesophageal manometry is also useful, but may occasionally be misleading, and an isotope emptying study (Figure 3.25) is a recent innovation which may be valuable in assessing therapy, although not necessarily diagnostic.

Management. The management of patients with achalasia has traditionally been by a Heller's myotomy. However, this necessitates a ten-day stay in hospital and in some patients a thoracoabdominal as opposed to an abdominal incision is required, thus increasing the surgical morbidity and mortality. Probably it should not now be the procedure of first choice in the elderly. The possibility of using pharmacology to influence the lower oesophageal sphincter has been considered and both calcium antagonists and nitrates can be tried. Isosorbide appears to be more beneficial than nifedipine, although with increased

Figure 3.24
a Barium swallow showing dilated oesophagus containing food debris and characteristic 'parrot's beak' deformity of lower oesophagus.
b Line drawing of the above.

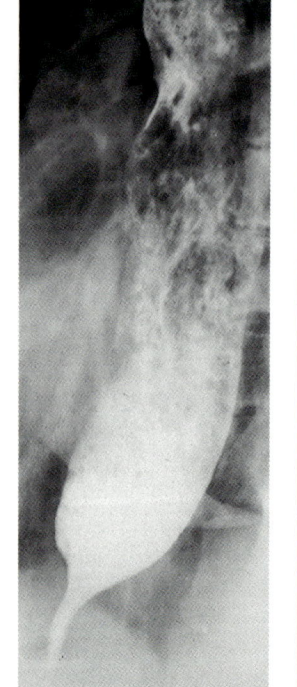

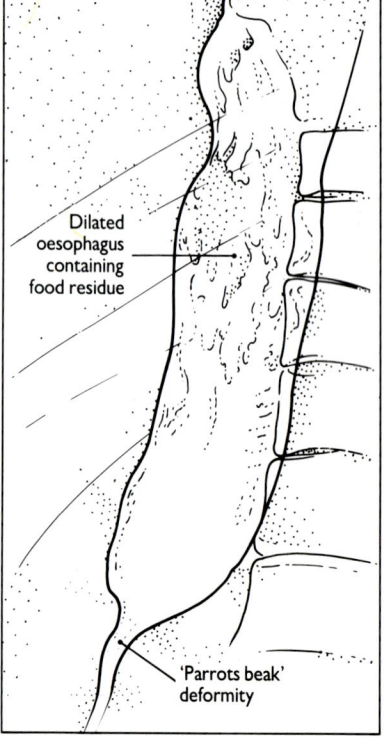

Figure 3.25
Oesophageal emptying study showing ingestion of radiolabelled test meal. Note extremely slow passage of the radiolabel into the stomach until ingestion of water at time 20 minutes.

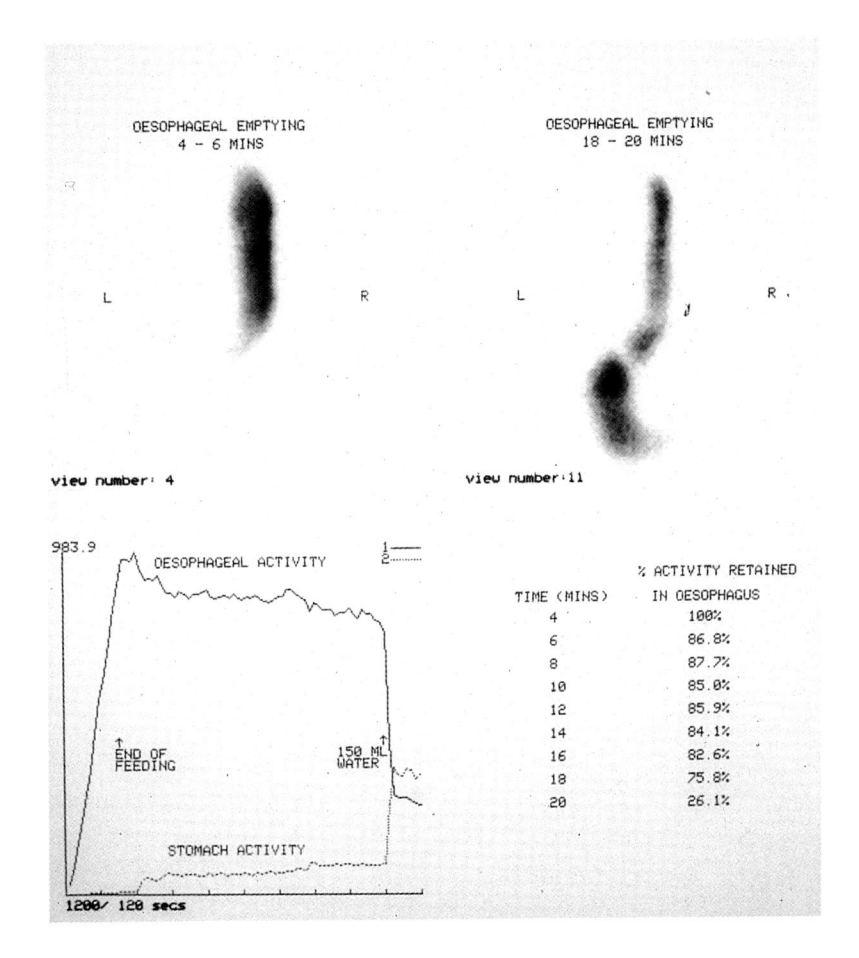

side-effects. Improvement by drugs may be only partially and temporarily effective. The recent use of forceful pneumatic balloon dilatation of the lower oesophageal sphincter would seem preferable in the elderly population, since it requires only an overnight stay in hospital. As with other endoscopic procedures, it can be performed under light intravenous sedation and 80-90% of patients will achieve full benefit after one, two or three dilatations at monthly intervals. In the long-term, both a Heller's myotomy and forceful pneumatic dilatation lead to an increased incidence of reflux, which can be troublesome. This risk appears to be greater after the surgical procedure. In this situation it is important that a standard antireflux operation is *not* performed, as this will only compound the swallowing difficulty.

Diffuse oesophageal spasm
This is an uncommon and difficult oesophageal problem, which occurs more frequently in the elderly population. Although bar-

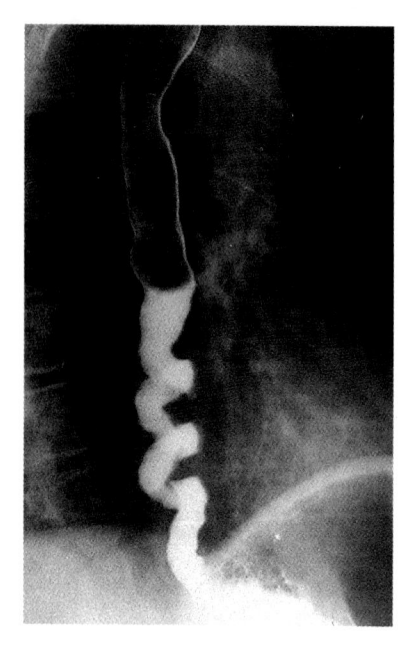

Figure 3.26
Plain x-ray showing tortuosity of the oesophageal lumen, a 'corkscrew oesophagus'.

ium x-rays may show marked oesophageal spasm (Figure 3.26), this does not necessarily correlate with symptoms. The symptoms of spasm are those of chest pain and dysphagia, sometimes induced by cold liquids.

Investigations are often unhelpful since spasm may not be present at the time of the test, and a normal barium x-ray will not exclude the diagnosis. Oesophageal manometry is therefore necessary to demonstrate the presence of high amplitude non-peristaltic contractions occurring in at least 30% of swallows. Although simple to perform and well tolerated by all age groups it is not widely available. Chest pain may mimic that of angina pectoris and indeed, spasm may be found in up to one-third of patients with chest pain who have normal coronary angiograms. Manometry demonstrates that the lower oesophageal sphincter pressure is normal in the majority of patients, although abnormal relaxation or elevated pressures may be seen in up to 30% of patients, some of whom may eventually evolve into classical achalasia.

The differentiation of oesophageal chest pain from that due to coronary artery disease can be extraordinarily difficult, and oesophageal disorders which can induce pain include reflux as well as achalasia and diffuse spasm. Due to the difficulties enumerated above in demonstrating spasm at a time of chest pain, provocation tests have been suggested including acid perfusion and the use of spasm-inducing agents such as edrophonium during manometry.

The use of ambulatory 24-hour pH monitoring using a direct recording pH sensitive nasogastric probe allows measurement of 24-hour distal oesophageal pH. Patients note any symptoms during this time and these can be correlated with the presence or absence of significant episodes of reflux.

Treatment with anticholinergic agents, calcium channel blockers (for example, nifedipine) or nitrates leads to a clinical improvement in a percentage of patients, and forceful pneumatic dilatation can be helpful in patients with abnormal lower oesophageal sphincter pressures. It has been sugggested that a long oesophageal myotomy may also be useful in intractable cases, but since this involves a thoracoabdominal incision elderly patients are usually not suitable. Nevertheless, there will remain a group of patients who undergo a gamut of investigations including exercise testing, coronary angiography, oesophageal manometry, pH recording, radiology and endoscopy, in whom a definitive diagnosis cannot be reached and who require symptomatic treatment on an empirical basis.

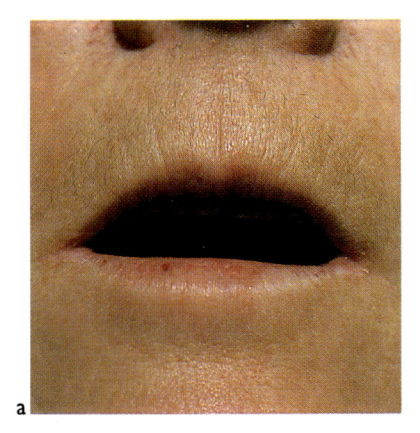

Figure 3.27
a Patient with systemic sclerosis showing a pinched mouth and lip telangiectases.
b Same patient's hands showing tight shiny skin over dorsum and hands.

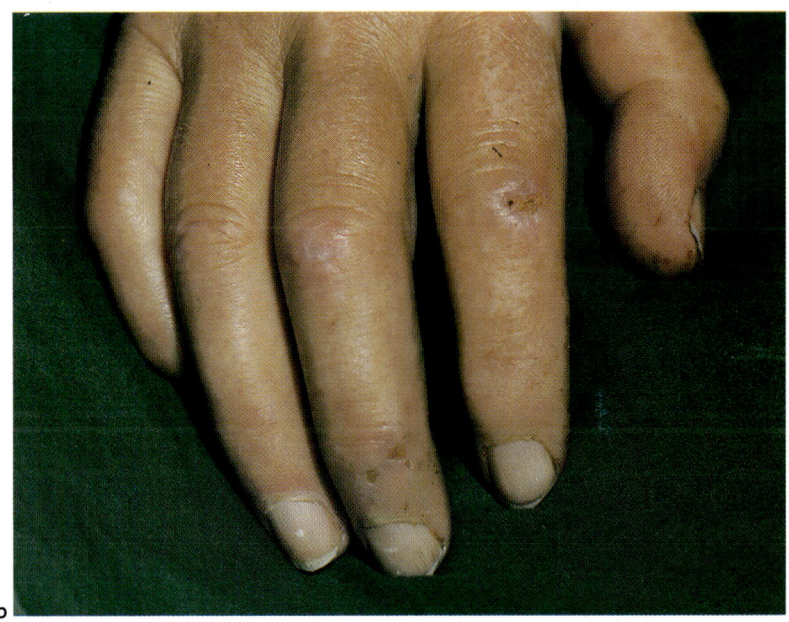

Progressive systemic sclerosis

In about 75% of patients with systemic sclerosis the oesophagus (Figure 3.27a and b) is involved. These patients have a marked diminution in peristaltic pressure in the distal two-thirds of the oesophagus and decreased lower oesophageal sphincter pressure. This in turn leads to severe reflux oesophagitis due to a combination of reflux and inability of the oesophagus to clear refluxed material back into the stomach. A similar picture may be seen in mixed connective tissue disease, and patients with systemic lupus erythematosus, idiopathic Raynaud's disease or dermatomyositis. Indeed, patients with Raynaud's phenomenon may have oesophageal dysfunction which predates the development of systemic sclerosis by several years.

Conclusions

A number of oesophageal problems are common in the elderly. Whilst many are benign they can be a source of much misery and a diminished quality of life. In general the age of the patient should not preclude adequate investigation since nearly all investigative procedures outlined in this chapter are well tolerated by even the frail and infirm. Subsequent appropriate management may be relatively simple but of immense benefit in relieving the patient's symptoms and in particular enjoyment of one of life's great pleasures, food and drink.

Bibliography

Richter JE, Castell DO. Gastro-oesophageal reflux, pathogenesis, diagnosis and therapy. *Annals of Internal Medicine.* 1982;**97**:93–103.

Editorial. Management of gastro-oesophageal reflux. *Lancet,* 1984;**i**:1054–1056.

Bennett J. A practical approach to reflux. *MIMS Magazine,* 1985;53–61.

Celestin LR, Campbell WB. A new and safe system for oesophageal dilatation. *Lancet,* 1981;**i**:74–75.

Ferguson R, Dronfield MW, Atkinson M. Cimetidine in treatment of reflux oesophagitis with peptic stricture. *British Medical Journal,* 1979;**2**:472–474.

Bozymski EM, Herlihy KJ, Orlando RC. Barrett's esophagus. *Annals of Internal Medicine,* 1982;**97**:103–107.

Heller SR, Fellows IW, Ogilvie AL, Atkinson M. Non-steroidal anti-inflammatory drugs and benign oesophageal stricture. *British Medical Journal,* 1982;**285**:167–168.

Hey H, Jorgensen F, Sorensen K, *et al.* Oesophageal transit of six commonly used tablets and capsules. *British Medical Journal,* 1982;**285**:1717–1719.

Mathieson R, Dutta SK. *Candida* esophagitis. *Digestive Diseases and Sciences,* 1983;**28**:365–370.

Boyce HW. Per oral prosthesis for palliating malignant esophageal and gastric obstruction. *Gastroenterology,* 1979;**77**:1141–1153.

Atkinson M, Ferguson R, Ogilvie AL. Management of malignant dysphagia by intubation at endoscopy, *Journal of the Royal Society of Medicine,* 1979;**72**:894–897.

Bennett JR. Intubation of gastro-oesophageal malignancies. *Gut,* 1981;**22**:336–338.

Earlam R, Cunha-Melo JR. Oesophageal squamous cell carcinoma: I. A critical review of surgery. *British Journal of Surgery,* 1980;**67**:381–390 II. A critical review of radiotherapy. *British Journal of Surgery,* 1980;**67**:457–461.

Cohen S. Motor disorders of the esophagus. *New England Journal of Medicine,* 1979;**301**:184–192.

Pelemans W, Vantrappen G. Oesophageal disease in the elderly. *Clinics in Gastroenterology*, 1985;**14**:635–656.

Lishman AH, Dellipiani AW. Management of achalasia of the cardia by forced pneumatic dilatation. *Gut*, 1982;**23**:541–544.

Bennett JR. Chest pain: heart or gullet? *British Medical Journal*, 1983;**286**:1231–1232.

Editorial. Angina and oesophageal disease. *Lancet*, 1986;**i**:191–192.

Gastro-duodenal disease in the elderly
R W Stockbrügger

The ageing of the stomach and duodenum

The study of age-related mucosal changes in the stomach and duodenum by post-mortem examination is unsatisfactory due to the destructive peptic effects of luminal contents. However, access to multiple biopsies obtained under visual control with highly-flexible fibre endoscopes has permitted some accurate scrutiny with a consequent increase in our knowledge of mucosal ageing. Although such investigative techniques may have become convenient, endoscopic biopsy studies on normal subjects of all ages are still rare.

Figure 4.1
Prevalence of gastritis in 155 persons selected at random

Fundic gastritis		45%
superficial		25%
atrophic		20%
(severe)		(6%)
Antral gastritis		68%
superficial		39%
atrophic		29%
Normal		22%

(Villako et al., 1976)

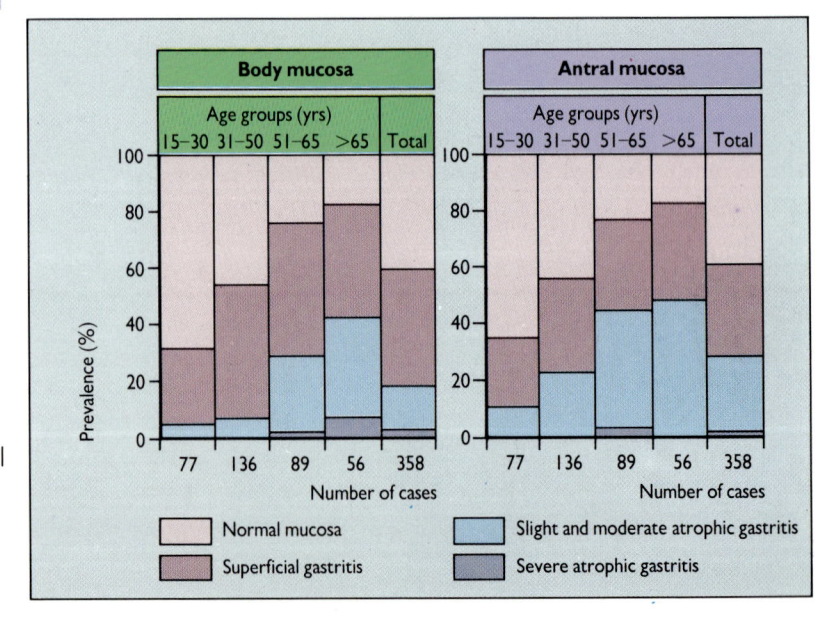

Figure 4.2
Biopsy findings of body and antral mucosa in a population sample representing a Finnish general population
(Siurala M et al. 1980)

As far as is known, only two studies exist in which the investigators have taken multiple duodenal and gastric biopsies from larger groups of healthy volunteers. The first one, from Estonia, comprised 155 individuals selected at random from a village population of 1059 subjects aged between 16 and 69 years. Among the volunteers, the male:female ratio was 38:62%, and the age distribution did not differ from that within the total population of the village (14.1% between 16 and 29 years, 39.5% between 30 and 49 years, 46.4% between 50 and 69 years).

The surprising result of this study was that the majority of the population had some form of gastritis with a high prevalence of atrophic gastritis (Figure 4.1) and the mucosal changes of the stomach increased with age (Figure 4.2).

The second study was part of a major research effort carried out by Siurala *et al.* in Finland to study the dynamics of chronic gastritis development. In a cross-sectional study and using a so-called stochastic mathematical model, they found a linear progression of antral gastritis which was similar in both sexes. Progression of fundal gastritis was, however, slightly different, as it started with a lower prevalence in young age groups and surpassed the frequency of antral gastritis at 60–70 years (Figure 4.3).

The progression of chronic gastritis, from superficial to severe atrophic form, has also been demonstrated by the same group in a long-term follow-up study.

Kreuning *et al.* studying gastric and duodenal mucosa in 50

Figure 4.3
Antrum and body age-dependent score (ADS) lines constructed from the Finnish family sample, females (F) and males (M) separately. Lines represent the mean progression of gastritis in the whole population sample. Note the initial higher ADS level in antrum but crossing-over of ADS lines at 60–70 years indicating more rapid progression of gastritis in the body in the population at large.

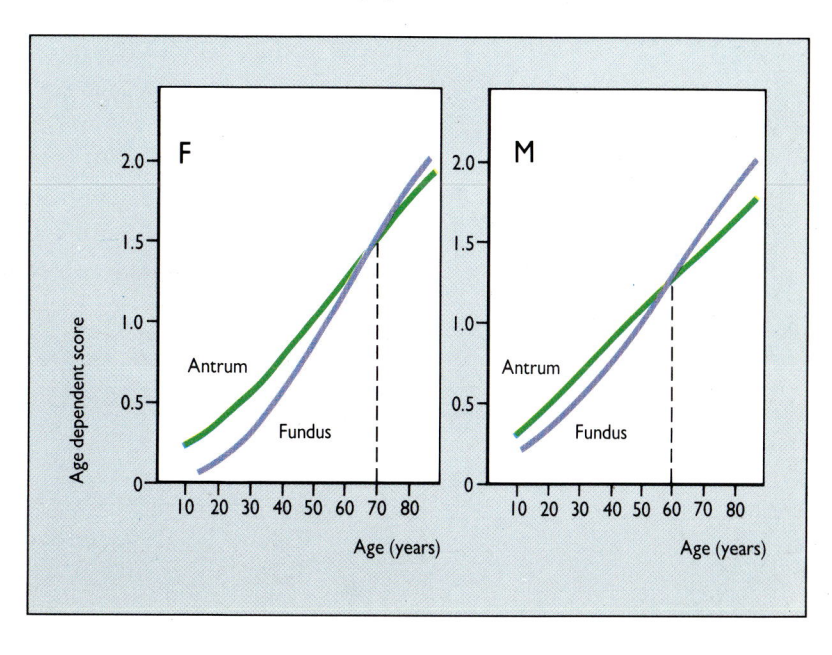

healthy volunteers, found gastritis in 18 (36%), and the likelihood increasing with age. They also found duodenitis in 12 volunteers (24%) but gave no age distribution for these cases.

Little is known about the morphological changes of the small-intestinal mucosa, but Holt has recently reviewed current knowledge of age-dependent changes in intestinal function. Appreciating the difficulties in studying nutrient absorption in elderly persons without disease, he concludes that there is no evidence for a decreasing capacity for fat, protein, or carbohydrate absorption with age in man. However, xylose absorption (that is the diffusion of a pentose) seems to diminish in very old age (above 80 years). Other studies have indicated that the absorption of iron and vitamin B_{12} is not impaired as a result of old age *per se*.

The development of atrophic gastritis

The stomach is divided into two morphologically different parts (Figure 4.4.). In the gastric antrum motor function is the main feature, but the mucosa also contains endocrine cells producing gastrin, somatostatin, and bombesin. The main function of the body/fundus of the stomach is storing, mixing, and chemically preprocessing nutrients before they are portioned out to the small bowel.

Preprocessing is achieved by hydrochloric acid and intrinsic factor produced by parietal cells, and by pepsin, produced by chief cells. Acid is needed for the sterilization of the bacterially contaminated food, and pepsin for a first step protein degradation. Intrinsic factor binds to vitamin B_{12} to secure the ileal absorption of this essential agent at an early stage.

Two main types of atrophic gastritis are described (Figure 4.5). In Type B the mucosal inflammation and atrophy ascends from the pyloric region along the lesser curvature. This type has little functional consequence as it rarely covers the greater parts of gastric body and fundus. It is quite common and is regarded as a

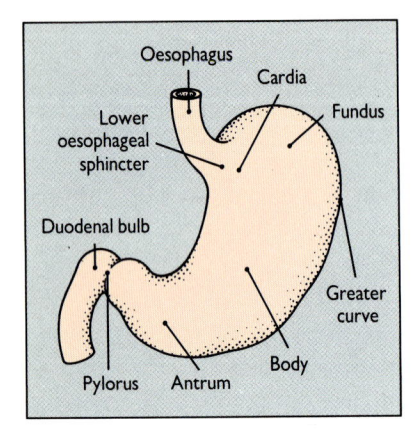

Figure 4.4
Morphologically and functionally the human stomach is divided into two parts 1) The antrum 2) The body/fundus.

Figure 4.5
Chronic atrophic gastritis.

Type A	Atrophy	body/fundus
	Gastrin	high
	Cause	endogenous/immunogenic
Type B	Atrophy	antrum/body/fundus
	Gastrin	normal
	Cause	exogenous/toxic

Figure 4.6
The endoscopic (left) and histological (right) appearance of severe mucosal atrophy in the gastric body area.

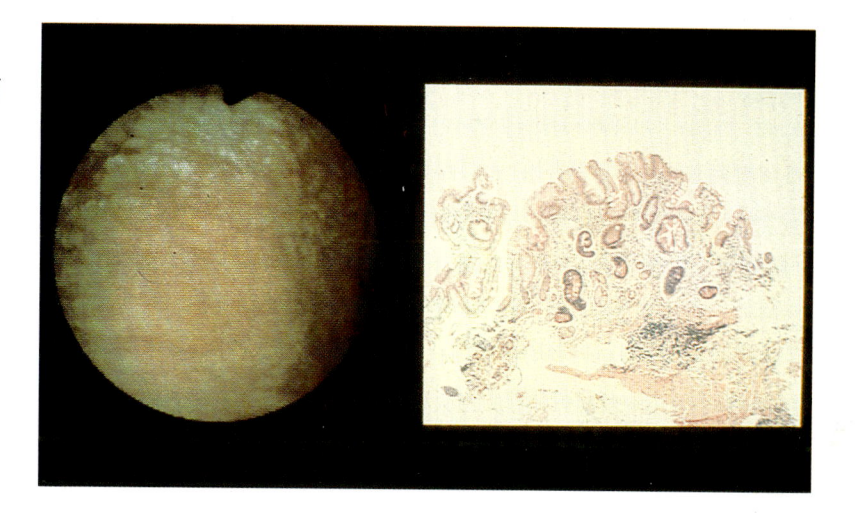

precancerous condition by some. Its causes are not established.

Atrophic gastritis of Type A has several important functional consequences, as it is localized in the body and fundus area, decreasing or abolishing the production of hydrochloric acid, intrinsic factor, and pepsin (Figure 4.6). Thus, it sometimes causes major clinico-pathological conditions, such as pernicious anaemia and bacterial overgrowth syndrome, which are dealt with elsewhere in this book.

Type A atrophic gastritis most probably has an immunological origin, as parietal cell and intrinsic factor antibodies are present in high frequency, and as it is associated with other autoimmune diseases, such as myxoedema, thyroiditis, Addison's disease, diabetes mellitus, and dermatitis herpetiformis.

Type A atrophic gastritis seems to be the principal morphological accompaniment to achlorhydria. It can sometimes be found in the young, but most often it is recognized in older age. Christiansen found achlorhydria in 4.7% of a normal population, and in 6.4% of patients with gastrointestinal symptoms. It was also significantly more frequent after the age of 60 years. Achlorhydria is not a pathological condition in itself and its presence should not be actively sought. However, once the diagnosis is made, future risk of pernicious anaemia and gastric malignancy should be remembered.

In achlorhydria, non-faecal and faecal bacteria are present not only in the luminal contents of the stomach and upper intestine, but also invading the mucosal layer. Bacterial overgrowth syndrome as a frequent cause of marginal or marked malabsorption in old age will be found in the chapter on malnutrition.

Vitamin B$_{12}$ deficiency and pernicious anaemia

Deficient intrinsic factor secretion is a consequence of atrophic gastritis affecting the body and fundus of the stomach. Intrinsic factor is still produced by remaining parietal cells even after hydrochloric acid secretion has ceased. The interval between the onset of achlorhydria and the drop in intrinsic factor production to a subnormal level varies with the individual. However, in a large series of patients with achlorhydric atrophic gastritis, Irvine *et al.* saw the development of vitamin B$_{12}$ malabsorption in 19% of 90 patients during a mean observation time of six years. Only two patients developed megaloblastic anaemia.

Vitamin B$_{12}$ deficiency does not occur only as a consequence of failure of intrinsic factor production or deficient absorption because of a diseased or resected distal ileum. It may also occur because of increased demand, for example, after acute blood loss or in chronic disease, precipitating an overt megaloblastic anaemia, or as a result of intraluminal consumption of the vitamin or the vitamin/intrinsic factor complex by gastrointestinal bacteria.

Pernicious anaemia is a disease of the elderly and the average age of onset is 60-70 years. It is recognized, when a macrocytic anaemia is found together with a megaloblastic bone marrow, low vitamin B$_{12}$ serum levels, and a positive Schilling test (less than 10% uptake of labelled vitamin B$_{12}$ and correction of absorption by addition of oral intrinsic factor). Pernicious anaemia is termed latent when all the previously mentioned features are found except the blood and bone-marrow findings (Figure 4.7).

Besides the haematological and neurological symptoms and signs of pernicious anaemia, the disease is of interest as it represents a so-called precancerous condition. It is uncertain, however, whether the atrophic changes in body and fundal mucosa alone, or their occurrence with a long-standing vitamin B$_{12}$ deficiency, are responsible for the three- to five-fold increase in gastric cancer risk.

The cancer risk in pernicious anaemia was difficult to assess while radiology, surgery, and post-mortems were the main dia-

Figure 4.7
Pernicious anaemia

Latent pernicious anaemia	Manifest pernicious anaemia
Gastric body mucosal atrophy	All features of latent pernicious anaemia plus:
Achlorhydria	
Low serum levels of vitamin B$_{12}$	macrocytic anaemia
Poor absorption of labelled vitamin B$_{12}$	megaloblastic bone marrow smear

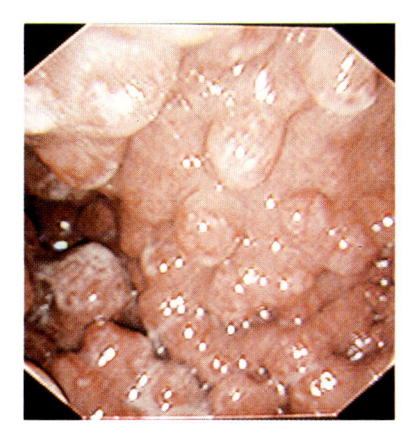

Figure 4.8
Endoscopic view of the body area of the stomach. Multiple 0.5 to 0.8 cm broadly based, polypoid lesions are visible.

gnostic methods for stomach diseases. A better assessment has been made recently by two major endoscopic screening studies. They established a prevalence of gastric cancer in correctly diagnosed and treated pernicious anaemia patients of 1.2% and 1.6% respectively. In addition, the studies showed a high prevalence of mild to severe dysplasia and frequent solitary or multiple micro-carcinoid tumours (Figures 4.8, 4.9 and 4.10).

Both studies included a follow-up or screening of patients over a period of 8 and 6 years, respectively, and showed no further instances of overt malignancy. Thus, the risk of developing a new gastric cancer after initial endoscopic screening is low and probably does not justify endoscopic examination of asymptomatic patients more frequently than approximately every five years.

As mentioned above, vitamin B_{12} deficiency is not only caused by deficient intrinsic factor production. In a large population study in Sweden, 293 persons aged 70 and 486 persons aged 75 were screened for serum vitamin B_{12} levels. In two consecutive tests subnormal values were found in 14 (4.8%) and 27 (5.6%), respectively. Of the 32 persons thoroughly investigated, only six had a latent (n=2) or manifest (n=4) pernicious anaemia. In the remaining 26, other causes were diagnosed or suspected (Figure 4.11). Surprisingly, in two patients consistently low values of serum vitamin B_{12} were found in the presence of duodenal ulcer, high acid secretion, and without signs of small bowel disease.

Figure 4.9
Gastric dysplasia and neoplasia in 80 patients with pernicious anaemia who had undergone gastroscopic screening in London 1978-1980

Dysplasia	
mild	24
moderate	6
severe	3
Polypoid lesions	18
Multiple APUD-cell tumours	1
Early gastric carcinoma	1

Figure 4.10
Dysplastic and neoplastic changes in 123 patients from central Sweden who had also undergone gastroscopic screening

Mild or moderate atypia in	11 (9%)
Non-polypoid mucosa	60 (49%)
Polypoid lesions	
hyperplastic/inflammatory	52
adenoma with moderate atypia	1
adenoma with early carcinoma	1
primary early adenocarcinoma	1
carcinoid tumour, solitary	4
carcinoid tumour, multiple	1

(according to Borch, 1986)

Figure 4.11
Causes of low vitamin B_{12} serum levels in 32 elderly patients who have undergone thorough gastroenterological investigation.

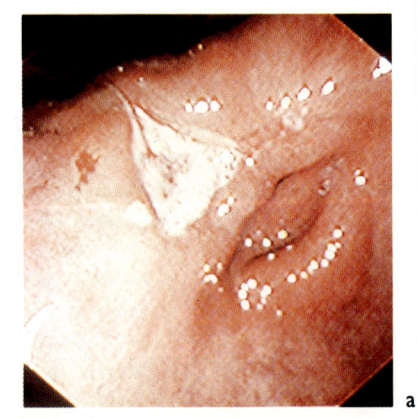

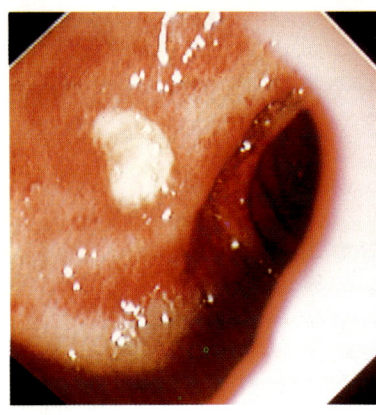

Figure 4.12
a Endoscopic view of benign gastric ulcer at the incisura of the stomach.
b Endoscopic view of duodenal ulcer.

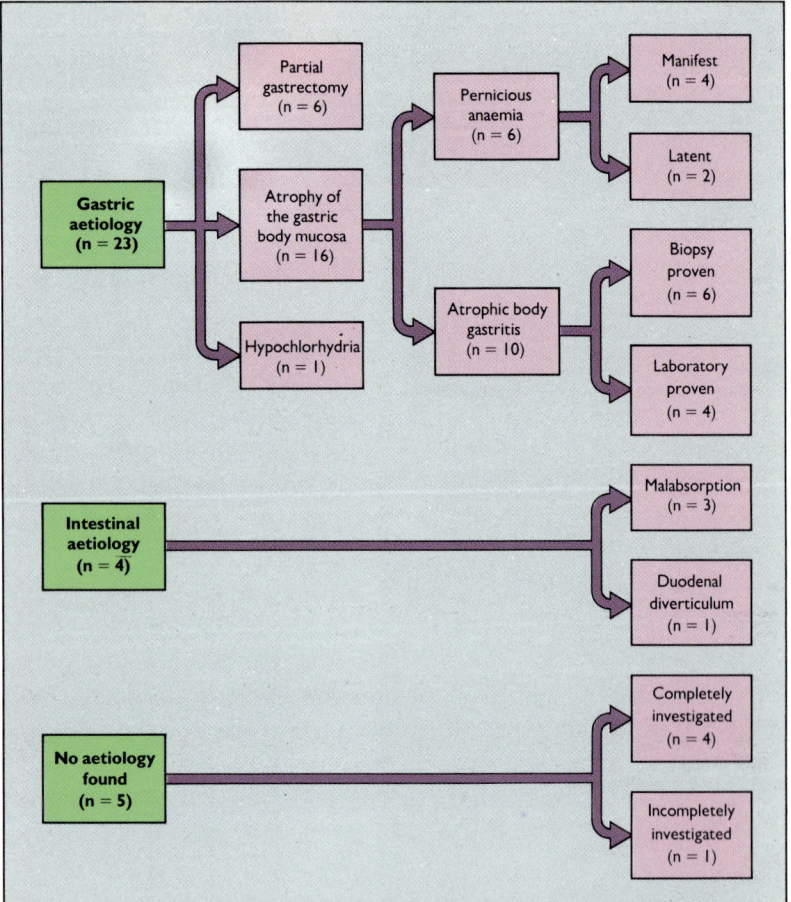

Duodenal and gastric ulcer in the elderly

Duodenal ulcer is not specifically a disease of the young and gastric ulcer is not a disease of the elderly (Figure 4.12). Both subcategories of peptic ulcer disease usually manifest themselves in middle age. In the famous epidemiological work of Bonnevie in Copenhagen, the average age at diagnosis of duodenal ulcer was 49 years and for gastric ulcer, 55 years, women being slightly older than men (Figures 4.13 and 4.14). The age-specific incidence of duodenal ulcer increases almost linearly up to the age of 75–79, where the incidence reaches 300 patients per 100,000 inhabitants per year. The same is true for gastric ulcer over the age of 40. In women of 70+ years, the ratio between duodenal ulcer and gastric ulcer is about 1:1 whereas for men it is about 2:1.

These figures are puzzling since it is known that gastric acid secretion decreases with increasing age. Thus, factors other than

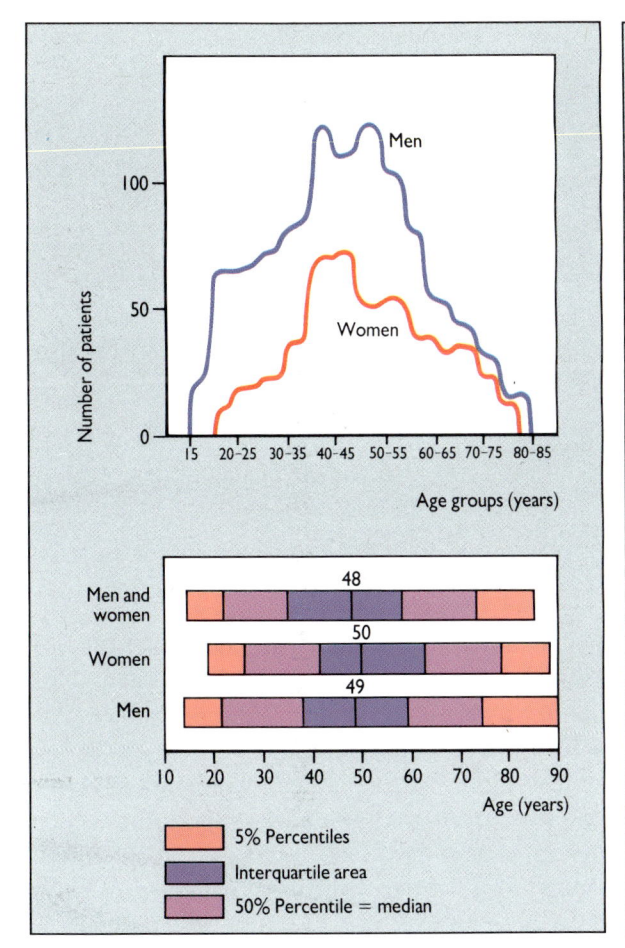

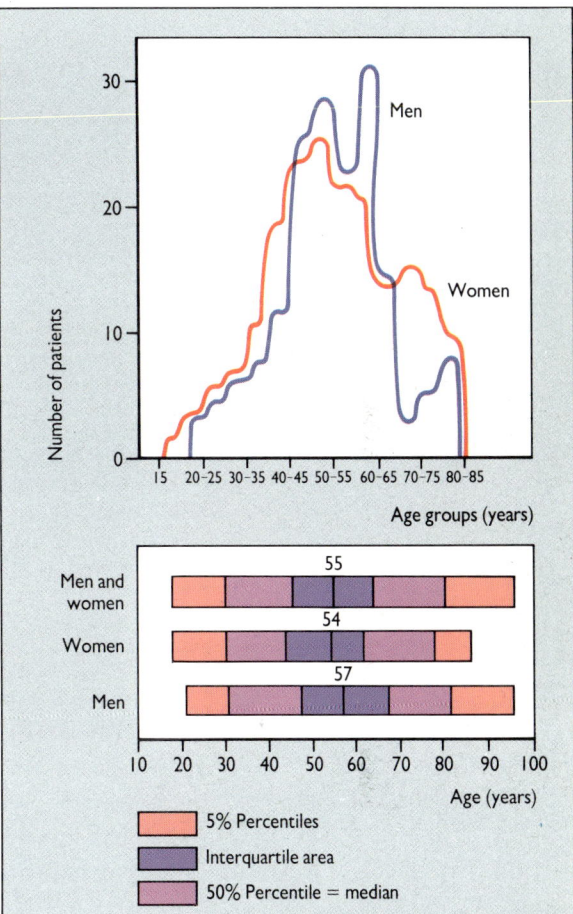

Figure 4.13 (left)
Patients with duodenal ulcer distributed according to age and sex
(Bonnevie)

Figure 4.14 (right)
Patients with solitary gastric ulcer distributed according to age and sex
(Bonnevie)

the quantity of acid secreted are important in the pathogenesis of peptic ulcer disease in the elderly and may also influence therapeutic considerations. Some of these factors have been recognized during the recent surge of interest in peptic ulcer disease initiated by access to endoscopy and potent pharmacological and surgical therapy.

One newly-recognized factor is cytoprotection or mucosal protection. These days, cytoprotection means not only a better or quicker repair of damaged or diseased superficial gastric epithelium, but also includes the whole process of mucosal regeneration or repair, involving such factors as cell turn-over, mucosal microcirculation, and scar formation (Figure 4.15). This process is partly directed by the paracrine and exocrine activity of mucosal prostaglandins.

For the elderly, the vascular component of this complex system may be particularly important. In extreme cases, large peptic

Figure 4.15
Theory of balance in the pathogenesis of peptic ulcer disease.

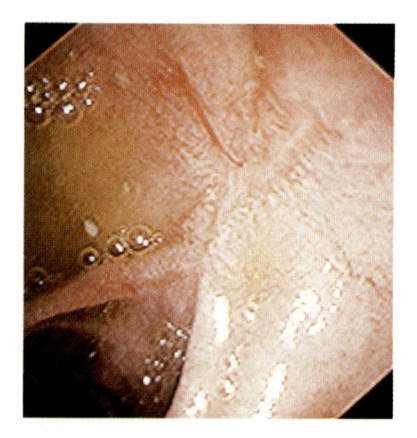

Figure 4.16
Scar in duodenal bulb of healed ulcer.

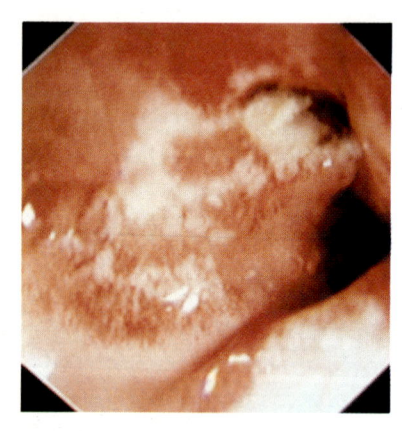

Figure 4.17
Deformation and active ulceration of duodenal bulb in a 72-year-old male patient with chronic peptic ulcer disease.

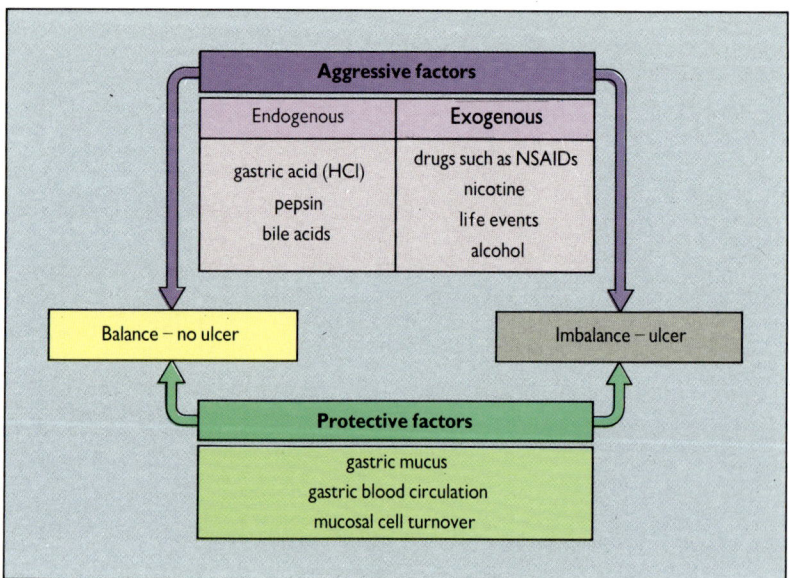

ulcers with atypical localization are found in patients with severe abdominal atherosclerosis. It is also conceivable, therefore, that minor deterioration in gastric blood flow may cause delayed ulcer healing or premature ulcer relapse in elderly patients. Within a mucosa with diffuse inflammatory and atrophic changes, the diminished reparative capacity may cause weak spots unprepared for the back diffusion of acid (although produced in normal or subnormal quantities) and subsequent ulcer formation.

Another factor in the pathogenesis of peptic ulcer disease in the elderly is the cumulative duodenal and gastric mucosal damage caused by repeated episodes of ulceration. Peptic ulcer disease is chronic and intermittent in many patients. Most ulcers will leave endoscopically visible or invisible scars (Figure 4.16). A more aggressive disease will cause severe deformations of the pyloric canal and duodenal bulb (Figure 4.17). The mucosa of these areas will not possess the same regenerative capacity as the mucosa in a patient presenting with an ulcer for the first time, and will be prone to further damage.

Apart from such intrinsic factors lowering gastric mucosal defence, one important extrinsic factor deserves discussion: non-steroidal anti-inflammatory drugs (NSAIDs). These drugs are frequently prescribed for the elderly and are often taken for non-specific symptoms originating from the musculoskeletal system. During a routine medical history such patients will rarely mention, or even remember, this form of drug intake, but closer questioning after endoscopic diagnosis of an ulcer or of diffuse

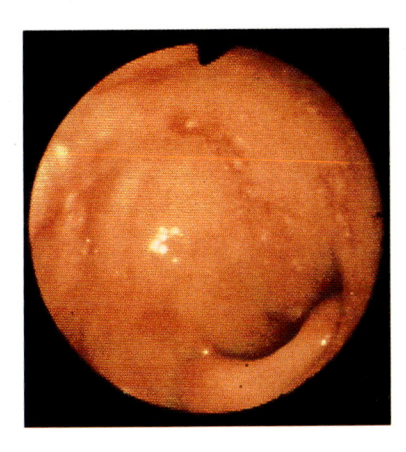

Figure 4.18
Haemorrhagic-erosive inflammation of the duodenal bulb in a patient on chronic NSAID treatment for rheumatoid arthritis.

haemorrhagic-erosive lesions will often reveal the noxious cause. Their association with peptic ulcer disease is well established (Figure 4.18).

Acid reduction and neutralization are certainly the first therapeutic measures to be taken against peptic ulcer disease in the elderly. The rationale of such treatment is not the elimination of excessive acid, but the reduction of the permissive acid factor, which is one of several factors in the pathogenesis of the ulcer disease.

However, improvement of mucosal defence is equally important: anaemia should be treated; smoking should be stopped; prescription and intake of non-steroidal anti-inflammatory drugs should be restricted to a necessary minimum. Recently published figures from Nottingham are a warning. The incidence and severity of peptic ulcer disease seems to be decreasing in the general population, but the incidence of emergency operations because of ulcer perforations in the elderly is rising.

It remains to be seen whether the cytoprotective factors can be administered or stimulated exogenously by drugs. It has been shown (though evidence is conflicting), that synthetic prostaglandin derivatives lead to better ulcer healing than their moderate acid-inhibitory effect would warrant. Cytoprotective properties are also attributed to various other anti-ulcer drugs, such as sucralfate, bismuth, and even aluminium-containing antacids (Figure 4.19).

Treatment of the elderly patient with peptic ulcer disease is in practice similar to that of younger patients. Duodenal ulcer(s) are, in most cases healed after a four- to six-week course with an H_2-antagonist. Healing need not necessarily be controlled by endoscopy; it can be assessed by the disappearance of symptoms.

Figure 4.19
Acid inhibition, mucosal protection and prevention of ulcer recurrence by various medical treatments

Gastric Mucosal Protection

Compound	Acid Inhibition	Mucosal Protection (Animal)	Mucosal Protection (Man)	Prevention of Recurrence
H_2 antagonists	+ +	0	0	0
Pirenzepine	+	+	(+)	0
Sucralfate	0	+ +	+ +	?
Bismuth subcitrate	0	+ +	+	?
Antacids, high dose	+ +	+ +	?	?
Antacids, low dose	+	+	(+)	?
Prostaglandins	+	+ +	(+)	0
Non-smoking	(+)	?	+	+

Gastric ulcer(s) should be managed in a different way (Figure 4.20). At the (obligatory) initial endoscopy the presence of malignancy has to be excluded by multiple biopsies from the ulcer base and margin. After a six- to eight-week course of H_2-antagonists, sucralfate, pirenzepine, or bismuth subcitrate, another endoscopy should be performed to check healing and obtain new biopsies, even from the ulcer scar.

Early and/or frequent recurrence of duodenal ulcer should raise suspicion of Zollinger-Ellison syndrome and this must be excluded by serial gastrin examinations before any decision on long-term treatment is made. When a gastric ulcer fails to heal or recurs quickly, dysplastic or malignant changes can often be found in subsequent biopsy or surgical specimens. Long-term medical treatment of gastric ulcer is therefore rather dubious. Surgical therapy within three to six months of the first diagnosis is recommended by most surgeons if a gastric ulcer fails to heal.

Duodenal ulcer is generally a benign condition, but complications, such as bleeding, perforation and gastric outlet obstruction occur with increasing frequency in the older age groups. The outcome of emergency measures in such situations is not without mortality. Therefore, continuous or intermittent long-term treatment with one of the above mentioned drugs should not be continued for longer than one or two years before elective surgery is taken into consideration.

The value of long-term therapy has been thoroughly evaluated only for H_2-antagonists and they should therefore be first choice, if long-term therapy is required. However, in the elderly they may cause confusion and can result in upper gastrointestinal bacterial overgrowth syndrome when pre-treatment gastric acid output is low.

The recently much-discussed *Campylobacter pylori* is not part of the bacterial overgrowth syndrome as it can be found in pre-treatment specimens from patients with gastric ulcer and chronic gastritis. Furthermore, *Campylobacter pylori* is not acid-sensitive and so far, it is doubtful whether *Campylobacter* retards ulcer heal-

Figure 4.20
Control of medical ulcer therapy

Duodenal ulcers	Gastric ulcers
initial endoscopy	initial endoscopy with multiple biopsies
control by symptoms	control-endoscopy after 6–8 weeks with new biopsies
re-endoscopy at relapse	
exclusion of Zollinger-Ellison syndrome	exclusion of malignancy
	surgical treatment to be considered after 3–6 months of non-healing

ing or causes early relapse. However, patients with non-healing ulcers in whom biopsy of the gastric antrum reveals strong growth of the bacteria should receive an antimicrobial agent.

One particular problem frequently encountered in geriatric gastroenterology is the necessity for NSAID treatment in spite of a pre-existing or subsequently occurring peptic lesion. Concomitant treatment with H_2-antagonists may reduce or even abolish the mucosal damage, but the ulcerogenic potency of the NSAID given may be stronger than the reparative effect of acid reduction. In such cases, a decision has sometimes to be made to withdraw NSAID. Unfortunately, no studies are yet published which indicate that prostaglandin analogues are better than H_2-antagonists in protecting against NSAID-induced lesions.

Gastric cancer

In recent decades a decline in gastric cancer mortality has been observed throughout many countries in spite of the increased life expectancy of the general population. The cause of this development is unknown but some data point to the effect of better food preservation (refrigeration instead of smoking and salting of foodstuffs) and to increased consumption of milk and vegetables. This hypothesis is supported by the fact that gastric cancer is still common in areas with poor living conditions and/or a relative lack of milk and vegetable products.

Medical advances may also help to mitigate the threat of this particular malignant condition. Access to endoscopic and preventive examinations for at-risk patients with precancerous conditions (for example, achlorhydric atrophic gastritis, post-gastrectomy stomach) has in some countries reduced the likelihood of early gastric cancer progressing to advanced malignancy.

However, gastric cancer is still high on the list of causes of death in the West and the average age at diagnosis is high. In a study from the Cleveland Clinic, the average age at diagnosis was 62 years; Borch *et al.* reported that 60% of their gastric cancer patients were 70+ years. It is twice as common in men as in women.

Gastric cancer in the elderly predominantly affects the antrum (about 50%), but a tendency to more proximal growth has recently been observed. It is mainly of the intestinal type and not of the more proliferative diffuse type according to the nomenclature of Lauren.

Symptoms of early gastric cancer are puzzling: epigastric pain, nausea, occasional vomiting, and weight loss are cited, but these

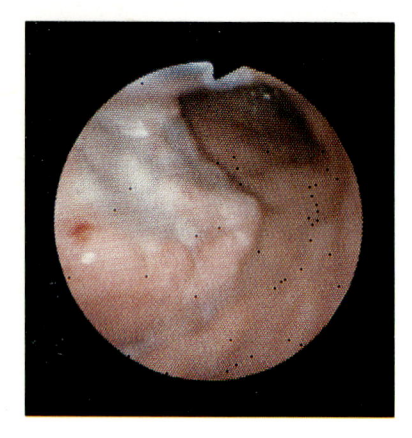

Figure 4.21
A large ulcerated area at the anterior wall of the stomach on the transition between the gastric antrum and body: an advanced adenocarcinoma of the intestinal type.

are also common complaints in the general population. If endoscopy is generally performed for these symptoms, a great deal of normal or less important findings will be obtained. However, in a screening study from Italy a high percentage of gastric carcinomas were diagnosed at an early stage.

Advanced gastric cancer may often involve major parts of the stomach without any symptoms, especially when it is present in the proximal stomach. Lesions involving the distal antrum and pyloric region may be diagnosed at an earlier stage because of symptoms associated with delayed gastric emptying.

Endoscopy is the best diagnostic technique for detection of gastric cancer (Figure 4.21). Paediatric instruments of 7 or 8 mm in outer diameter in combination with mild sedating medication render endoscopy highly tolerable in trained hands (Figure 4.22). The elderly patient is usually more relaxed during endoscopy than a young, nervous (and often cigarette-abusing) patient. In the course of the examination, multiple biopsies are easily taken from all suspicious lesions. In a recent study in Munich by Ottenhann, 8% of the endoscopically-diagnosed gastric ulcers were found to be malignant on histology (Figure 4.23).

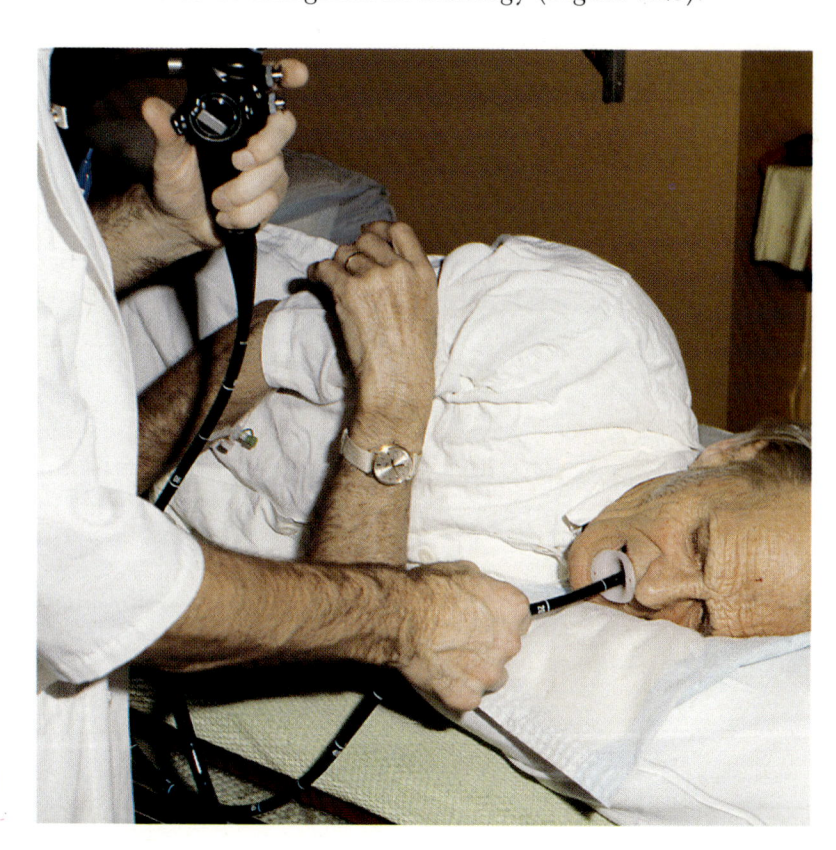

Figure 4.22
Upper gastrointestinal-endoscopy is very well tolerated even in old age.

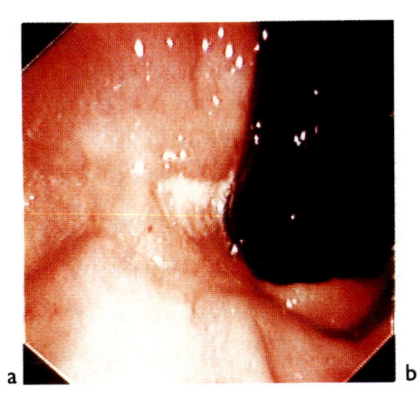

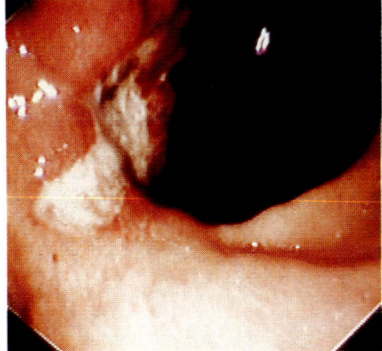

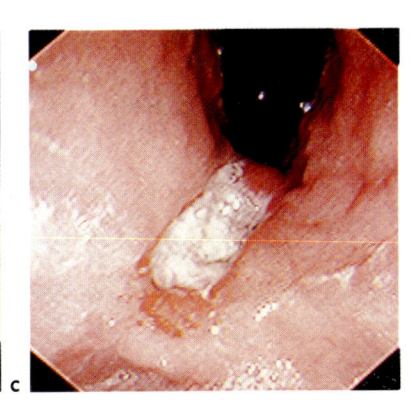

Figure 4.23
a to c Three endoscopic views of gastric ulcers which were shown histologically to be malignant. At endoscopy these ulcers were thought likely to be benign.

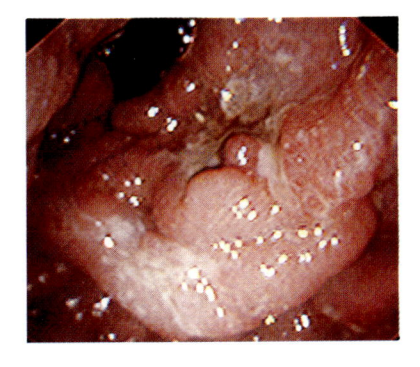

Figure 4.24
Endoscopic view of lymphomatous infiltration of the body and fundus of the stomach visualized by endoscopic retroversion.

Figure 4.25
a Endoscopic view of the antrum of the stomach showing slight mucosal irregularity.
b Biopsy of this area was reported as consistent with early gastric cancer.

Surgery is currently the only possible means of curing gastric malignancy whether a carcinoma or lymphoma (Figure 4.24). Five-year survival rates may be as high as 95% in early gastric carcinoma (Figure 4.25). In advanced cancer it is considerably less, but recently improved by better anaesthetic and surgical techniques. In the tumour centre at Erlangen in West Germany, five-year survival rose significantly from 23% to 32% within ten years. Subtotal or total gastrectomy are the operations of choice. Extended dissection of perisplenar and para-aortic lymph nodes has been employed at some leading centres.

Quality of life after total gastrectomy has previously been considered to be poor. In our own group of 11 patients aged 63–83 years (average 70 years) with no signs of recurrent disease the average body weight was subnormal in nine patients with an average deficit of 5.6 kg. They all had steatorrhoea, from 102 to 468 mmol fatty acids per 72 hours (upper normal limit 60 mmol per 72 hours). In contrast to these objective findings, very few digestive or other complaints were expressed postoperatively by these patients. It was interesting that only six out of eleven had a short oro-caecal transit time (below 120 min), as measured by

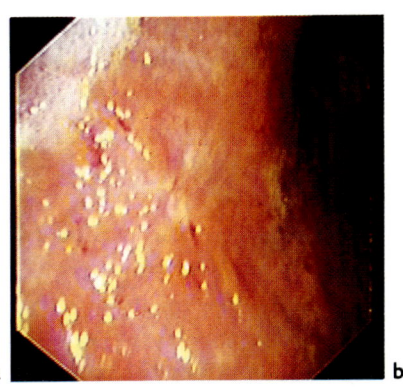

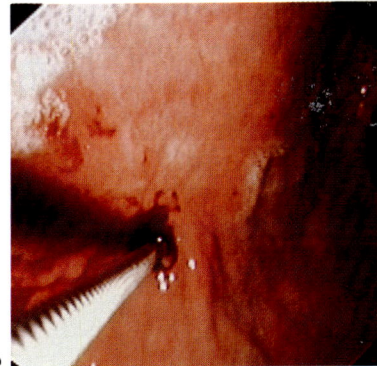

Figure 4.26
The predominant symptoms in 83 adult patients with coeliac disease

Diarrhoea and weight loss	71
Constipation	1
Anaemia	7
Oedema	1
Epigastric pain	3

(Gillberg, 1981)

Figure 4.27
Pathological, laboratory testing in adult patients with coeliac disease

Steatorrhoea	58/64	91%
Xylose absorption test	56/63	89%
Plasma folate	41/62	66%
Blood folate	38/58	66%
Lactose tolerance test	32/52	62%
Low serum vitamin B_{12}	22/65	34%

(Gillberg 1981)

the hydrogen breath test, in spite of the fact that the storage function of the stomach had been abolished by the operation.

In gastric cancer, extended surgery should be undertaken only if there is a reasonable chance of cure. Large palliative measures do not prolong life, and may actually decrease the quality of the remaining life-span. Further, they necessitate prolonged health care and can often be replaced by enteral or parenteral nutrition and generous analgesia.

Diffuse and localized mucosal changes of the duodenum

Gluten-induced enteropathy (coeliac disease) is a disease traditionally associated with childhood. Nevertheless, during the last decade it has also been recognized in the middle-aged and elderly. In a study reported by Swinson *et al.*, 25% of the patients were aged over 60 at the time of the diagnosis.

It remains uncertain, however, whether this finding of coeliac disease in the elderly is real or caused by improved diagnosis of patients with minor symptoms and signs. There is considerable support for the latter hypothesis. Swinson *et al.* found that only 26% of their patients suffered from severe anaemia, osteomalacia, or steatorrhoea. The clinical picture was similar in a Swedish study by Gillberg *et al.*, in which diarrhoea and weight loss were the most frequent symptoms of coeliac disease (Figure 4.26) and steatorrhoea, xylose malabsorption and folate deficiency the most frequent laboratory findings (Figure 4.27). Low blood folate and diminished xylose absorption are sensitive markers of coeliac disease.

Diagnostic procedures for coeliac disease have become less demanding on the patient. Instead of several malabsorption tests followed by a capsule biopsy from the upper jejunum, nowadays an upper gastrointestinal-endoscopy with multiple biopsies from the second part of the duodenum provides adequate sampling of the small intestinal mucosa. The diagnostic congruence of multiple small duodenal and one large jejunal biopsy has been demonstrated by several workers.

Unfortunately therapy has not changed in the same favourable way as diagnosis, and still consists of a strict gluten-free diet with a risk of relapse after minor dietary lapses or sins. The elderly patient certainly has as many difficulties in adhering to the prescribed diet as the child with coeliac disease. A change in eating habits after many years of habituation is always a problem which is also evident in other metabolic diseases such as diabetes or

Figure 4.28
Histological grading of duodenitis

Grade of duodenitis	Distinguishing histological features	General histological features
0	normal	neutrophil polymorph infiltration + or − increasing cellularity of lamina propria and loss of villous surface pattern metaplasia + or −
1	superficial epithelium and general morphology normal increased cellularity of lamina propria	
2	abnormality of the surface epithelium	
3	erosion of the surface epithelium	

(Whitehead, 1975)

Figure 4.29
Pathological findings in the duodenum at an endoscopic survey of 80 patients with pernicious anaemia

Duodenitis	35
mild	33
moderate	2
Partial villous atrophy	6
malignant cells	1

(Stockbrügger et al 1983)

obesity and the minor degree of symptoms contributes to lack of motivation. In addition, gluten-free cereals may be difficult to obtain, and even if home-made the taste of gluten-free bread remains, at best special.

Villous atrophy is not only found in coeliac disease or tropical sprue but may also be seen in non-specific severe duodenitis to a marked degree (Figure 4.28). Non-specific duodenitis may be localized or general.

Bulbar duodenitis often accompanies duodenal ulcer and can also be seen in the pre- or post-ulcer phase. It can be recognized endoscopically by redness, friability, or small erosive and haemorrhagic changes. Treatment is the same as for duodenal ulcer disease in symptomatic cases.

More generalized duodenitis has recently been described in patients with achlorhydria and pernicious anaemia, in association with partial villous atrophy (Figure 4.29) or lymphonodular infiltration (Figure 4.30). As most of these patients had gastroduodenal growth of faecal-type bacteria, it seems reasonable to link the mucosal changes to the altered intraluminal flora. The patients with achlorhydria and duodenitis had symptoms and signs of impaired absorption unlike those with achlorhydria and no duodenitis. Whether this difference is due to the mucosal alterations, to the bacterial interference, or to a combination of both remains to be elucidated.

Other diffuse mucosal changes of the duodenum are rare. In patients with severe systemic disease the possibility of amyloido-

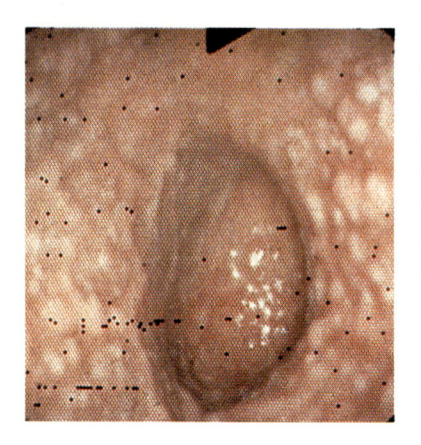

Figure 4.30
The duodenal bulb contains multiple white lesions of the size of the head of a pin. Histologically enlarged lymphatic folliculi.

Figure 4.31
Multiple aphthous lesions of the second part of the duodenum: Crohn's disease.

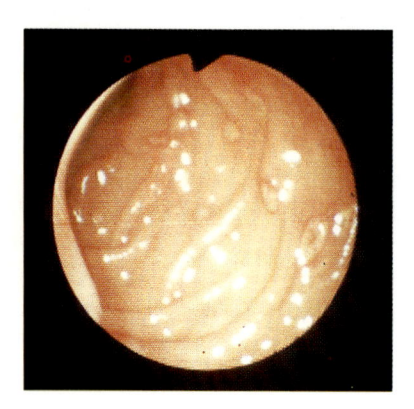

Figure 4.32
Numerous *Giardia lamblia* in a smear from the mid-duodenum obtained by endoscopic brush cytology.

sis should be considered. The rare elderly patient with Crohn's disease may present with duodenal manifestations (Figure 4.31). Drug-induced damage of the duodenum and upper jejunum has become infrequent since the introduction of slow-release preparations for potassium supplementation of diuretic therapy. Giardiasis with malabsorption and/or diarrhoea is certainly still underdiagnosed and is not only found in patients who have travelled abroad. It may easily be missed when only stool specimens are examined (although these may have been freshly obtained), but is most efficiently diagnosed by careful microscopy of duodenal biopsies (Figure 4.32).

Duodenal diverticula

Unfortunately, there are no hard data about the prevalence of duodenal diverticula in general, or in particular in the elderly. Thus we do not know, whether incidence increases with age, as is the case for colonic diverticula. Duodenal diverticula are demonstrated in 2% of radiological examinations. They are most frequently localized in the second (descending) part of the duodenum (Figure 4.33). Probably they are underdiagnosed by routine barium examination; pharmacological relaxation of the duodenum during radiological examination, and duodenoscopy may mean that they are identified more frequently.

Duodenal diverticula have recently gained clinical importance for two related reasons. Firstly, even if small, diverticula make

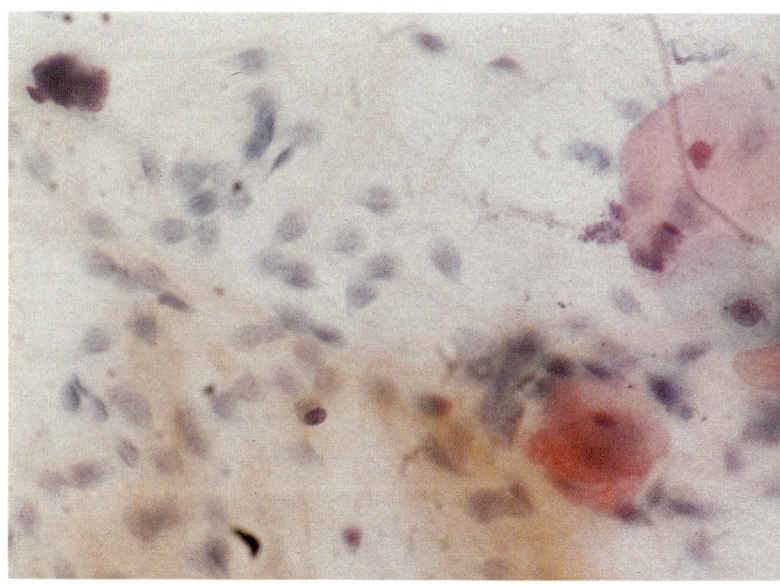

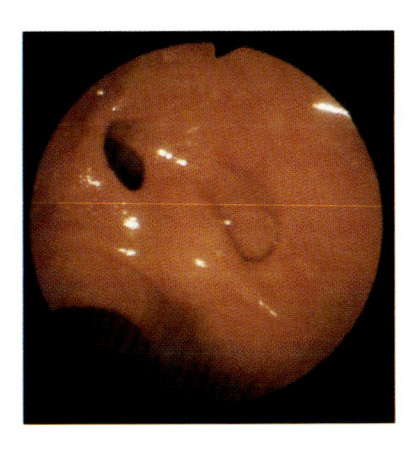

Figure 4.33
Two diverticula, one deep and one shallow, close to the ampulla of Vater.

up a blind loop harbouring undigested sludge which is bacterially contaminated particularly when gastric acid secretion is low or absent. They may cause malabsorption.

Secondly, when diverticula are localized close to the papilla of Vater (juxtapapillary) (Figures 4.34 and 4.35), or when the papilla is localized within the diverticulum, they are associated with an increased risk of biliary disease (cholangitis, cholecystitis, recurrent bile duct stones after cholecystectomy). They are believed to cause biliary disease by lowering biliary sphincter tone, allowing bacteria to ascend from the duodenum. The presence of bacteria in the bile duct may result in crystallization of bile and the formation of biliary sludge and stone.

Treatment of the latter condition may be difficult, as surgical intervention is often impossible or hazardous. An endoscopic sphincterotomy sometimes provides the solution, but cannot be performed with the papilla at the bottom of a deep diverticulum. Medical treatment should concentrate on the bacterial contamination, and will consist of repeated courses of antibiotics. In the case of gastric hyposecretion, the value of frequent acidification of the stomach and duodenum by acidic beverages (fresh lemonade; acid-containing soft drinks) has not been documented scientifically, but has been beneficial in some of our patients.

Conclusion

Gastroduodenal disease of the elderly is of great importance in general practice as well as in hospital care. A good knowledge of the similarities with and differences in the disease spectrum of younger age groups is therefore essential.

First of all, it has to be remembered that a number of pathological gastroduodenal conditions occur predominantly in advanced age, for example, achlorhydric atrophic gastritis, with or without pernicious anaemia, and gastric cancer. In other conditions, for example, gastric ulcer, the average age of onset is certainly below 65 years, but the age range is very wide and includes the very old. In addition, some disease entities believed to be prevalent only in the young are now also diagnosed in older age groups with increasing frequency.

Although the clinical picture of gastroduodenal disease of the elderly is principally similar to that of younger age groups, with increasing age the problem of concurrent disease and consequences of medical and previous surgical treatment may overshadow typical symptoms or signs of a newly-developed condition.

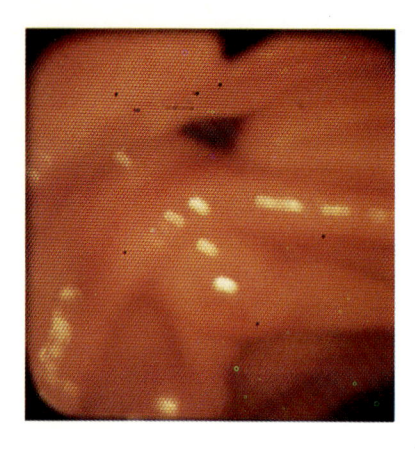

Figure 4.34
The orifice of a large juxtapapillary diverticulum which has caused recurrent cholangitis in an elderly woman.

Fortunately, investigation of gastroduodenal disease is relatively easy in elderly patients: contraindications to upper gastrointestinal endoscopy are rare. This investigation will provide direct evidence of most diseases in the area, especially when inspection is combined with pH measurement, sampling of gastroduodenal juice for microbial culture, and multiple biopsies.

Diagnostic achievements are only of real value when they can be followed by therapeutic measures. Nowadays, medical treatment of, for example, peptic ulcer disease is nearly as efficient for the elderly as for the young age groups. However, the side-effects of medication become manifest mainly in older age groups, for example, mental symptoms after H_2-antagonists. Surgery for malignant disease still carries a high risk in the elderly despite improvements in surgical and anaesthetic techniques.

Therefore, early diagnosis and preventive investigation of precancerous states (such as tubular adenomas of the colon) and precancerous conditions (such as pernicious anaemia) are to be recommended with the aim of avoiding a late diagnosis of an advanced disease in old age.

Bibliography

Villako K *et al.* Prevalence of antral and fundic gastritis in a randomly selected group of an Estonian rural population. *Scandinavian Journal of Gastroenterology*, 1976;**11**:817–822.

Siurala M *et al.* New aspects on epidemiology, genetics and dynamics of chronic gastritis. *Frontiers in Gastrointestinal Research*, 1980;**6**:148–166.

Siurala M *et al.* Long term follow-up of subjects with superficial gastritis or a normal gastric mucosa. *Scandinavian Journal of Gastroenterology*, 1971;**6**:459–463.

Kreuning J *et al.* Gastric and duodenal mucosa in 'healthy' individuals. *Journal of Clinical Pathology*, 1978;**31**:69–77.

Holt PR. The small intestine. *Clinics in Gastroenterology*, 1985;**14** (no 4):689–724.

Christiansen PM. Aklorhydri hos voksne. Copenhagen 1970. P. Hansens Bogtrykkeri:*Munksgaard*.

Irvine WJ *et al.* Natural history of autoimmune achlorhydric atrophic gastritis A 1–15 year follow-up study. *Lancet*, 1974;**ii**:482–485.

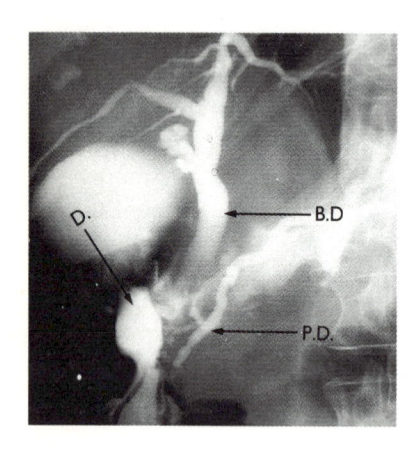

Figure 4.35
X-ray taken during ERCP showing pancreatic duct (PD), bile duct (BD) and diverticulum (D) as shown in Figure 4.34.

Stockbrügger R *et al*. Gastroscopic screening in 80 patients with pernicious anaemia. *Gut*, 1983;**24**:1141–1147.

Borch K. Epidemiologic, clinicopathologic and economic aspects of gastroscopic screening of patients with pernicious anaemia. *Scandinavian Journal of Gastroenterology*, 1986;**21**:21–30.

Nilsson-Ehle *et al*. Low serum cobalamin levels in a population study of 70 and 75-year-old subjects. Gastrointestinal causes and hematological effects. *Digestive Diseases and Sciences*, 1988 (in press)

Diehl JT *et al*. Gastric carcinoma. A 10 year review. *Annals of Surgery*, 1983;**198**:9–12.

Borch K *et al*. Gastric cancer. Diagnosis, treatment and prognosis in clinical routine. *Acta Chirurgica Scandinavica*, 1982;**148**:517–523.

Lauren P. The two histological main types of gastric carcinoma: diffuse and so-called intestinal type carcinoma. *Acta Pathologica Microbiologica Scandinavica*, 1965;**64**:31–49.

Crespi M. *et al*. The diagnosis of the carcinoma of the stomach in its early phase. *Archives Françaises des Maladies de l'Appareil Digestif*, 1972;**61**:285.

Swinson CM *et al*. Is coeliac disease underdiagnosed? *British Medical Journal*, 1980;**281**:1258–1260.

Gillberg R. Causes of malabsorption after total gastrectomy with Roux-en-y reconstruction *Thesis* 1981, Goteborg, Sweden.

Gillberg R *et al*. Coeliac disease diagnosed by means of duodenoscopy and endoscopic duodenal biopsy. *Scandinavian Journal of Gastroenterology*, 1977;**12**:911–916.

Stockbrügger RW *et al*. Pernicious anaemia, intragastric bacterial overgrowth and possible consequences. *Scandinavian Journal of Gastroenterology*, 1984;**19**:355–364.

Index

Achalasia, cardia, 51–53
  aetiology, 51
  diagnosis, 51
  investigations, 52
  management, 52–53
Achlorhydria in atrophic gastritis, 61, 62
  and duodenitis, 73
ACTH-producing tumours, oral pigmentation, 30
Acyclovir tablets in the *Herpes zoster* infection, 23
Addison's disease, buccal pigmentation, 30
Adenocarcinoma, cardio-oesophageal junction, 45
  oesophageal, 48
Ageing of cells, 12–13
  duodenum, 58–64
  and population growth, 8–9
  stomach, 13–14, 58–64
  and treatment advances, 9–10
Agranulocytosis, oral ulceration, 26
Alginic acid in oesophageal reflux, 39
Amphotericin-B in infective oesophagitis, 43–44
Amyloidosis and duodenal mucosal changes, 73–74
Anaemia, oral ulceration, 26
  see also Pernicious anaemia
Antrum
  and body age-dependent score, 59
  in gastric cancer, 70, 71
Aphthous ulceration, recurrent, 20–21
  treatment, 21
Atrophic gastritis *see* Gastritis, atrophic

Bacterial overgrowth syndrome, 68
Barium studies
  in achalasia of the cardia, 52
  in infective oesophagitis, 43
  oesophageal carcinoma, 47
  in oesophageal reflux, 36–38
  in pharyngeal pouch, 50
  showing oesophageal stricture, 40
Barrett's oesophagus complicating oesophageal reflux, 42
  endoscopy, 42
  management, 42
Bed occupancy according to age, 9–10
Behçet's syndrome, oral ulceration, 21, 26
  characteristics, 26
  management, 26
Benzocaine in aphthous ulcers, 21
Benzydamine in aphthous ulcers, 21
Betamethasone valerate pellets in lichen planus, 24
Bile duct disorders, 15
Black hairy tongue, 33
Bullae, oral, 30–32

Campylobacter pylori, bismuth-containing agents, 14
  and ulcers, 68–69
Cancer, gastrointestinal tract, deaths, 16
  see also specific regions
Candida, on lichen planus, tongue, 25
  and oesophagitis, 43
Candidiasis, oral, 21–22
  causing plaque, 29
Carbenoxylone sodium in aphthous ulcers, 21

Cardia, achalasia, 51–54
  see also Achalasia
Carmelose sodium in aphthous ulcers, 21
Celestin dilator, 41
Cells, ageing, 12–13
Chlorhexidine mouthwash for aphthous ulceration, 21
Cholangitis and bile duct disorders, 17
Cimetidine, introduction, 11
Cirrhosis and plaque, 29
13-Cis-retinoic acid in leukoplakia, 28
Coeliac disease, 72
  diagnostic procedures, 72
  predominant symptoms, 72
Colonic cancer, 16
  survival, 18
Colonoscopy, tolerance, elderly, 17
Crohn's disease, oral stomatitis, 27
Cytoprotection in ulcer disease, 65, 66, 67

Dietary deficiency and oral ulceration, 27
Dietary factors causing disease, 13
Diffuse oesophageal spasm, 53–54
  differential diagnosis, 54
  investigations, 54
  management, 54
  symptoms, 53
Dilatation, balloon, in achalasia of the cardia, 53, 54
Dilators, oesophageal, 41
Diverticula, oesophageal, 41
Diverticula, duodenal, 74–75
  clinical features, 74–75
  investigations, 74
  treatment, 75

Drug-induced
  duodenal damage, 74
  erythema multiforme, 24
  lichen planus, 24
  mouth ulcers, 21
  oesophagitis, 42–43
  oral pigmentation, 30
  oral ulceration, 21
Duodenal ulcer, 64–69
  acid inhibition, 67
  bulb, 66
  Campylobacter pylori, 68
  complications, 68
  endoscopy, 12
  epidemiology, 64–65
  mucosal protection, 65, 66, 67
  NSAIDs, 66
  pathogenesis, 66
  prevention of recurrence, 67
  treatment, 67, 68
  Zollinger-Ellison syndrome, 68
Duodenitis
  and achlorhydria, 73
  bulbar, 73
  grading, 73
  and pernicious anaemia, 73
Duodenum
  ageing, 58–64
  diverticula, 74–75
    see also Diverticula
  mucosal changes, 58
    biopsy investigations, 59
Dysphagia
  in achalasia of the cardia, 51
  in oesophageal carcinoma, 46
  oropharyngeal, 49

Eder Puestow olives, 41
Elderly, proportion in population, 9
Endoscopes, advent, 11
Endoscopy in
  achalasia of the cardia, 52
  atrophic gastritis, 61
  Barrett's oesophagus, 42
  duodenal diverticula, 75
  duodenal ulcer, 12
  gastric cancer, 70
  gastric ulcer, 68
  oesophageal carcinoma, 47
  oesophageal reflux, 38, 40–41
    sedation, 41
  pernicious anaemia, duodenum, 73
Erythema multiforme, 24–25
  drugs inducing, 24
  vulval/urethral complications, 25
Erythroplasia, 29

Faecal incontinence, management, 18

Gastric cancer, 69–72
  advanced, 70
  causes, 69
  endoscopy, 70
  incidence, 69
  surgery, 71
    quality of life after, 71–72
  symptoms, 69–70
Gastric ulcer, 64–69
  acid inhibition, 67
  benign high lesser curve, 14
  epidemiology, 64–65
  mucosal protection, 65, 66, 67
  NSAIDs, 66
  pathogenesis, 66
  prevention of recurrence, 67
  treatment, 67, 68
Gastritis
  antral, 59
  atrophic, achlorhydria, 61, 62
    associated disorders, 61
    development, 60–61
    endoscopy, 61
    prevalence, 59
    types, 60–61
  chronic, 59
    progression, 59
    mucosal changes, 59
    prevalence, 59, 60
Gastro-duodenal disease, elderly, 58–77
Gastrointestinal bleeding (haemorrhage), 11
  in infective oesophagitis, 43
  reduction, and endoscopy, 14–15
Geographic tongue, 33
Giardiasis and duodenal mucosal changes, 74
Gingival hypertrophy, 31–32
Gingivitis, acute ulcerative, management, 21
Glossitis, 32
Gold therapy and soft palate ulcers, 21
Granulomatosis, Wegener's, 27

H_2 receptor antagonists (H_2 blockers), 11–12, 14
  in duodenal ulcer, 68
  in oesophageal reflux, 39, 40
  in peptic ulcer disease, 14
Halitosis, 20, 32
  causes, 32
  and systemic disorders, 32

Heller's myotomy in achalasia of the cardia, 52
Herpes simplex and oesophagitis, 43, 44
Herpes zoster, oral, 23
  Acyclovir, 23
  post-herpetic neuralgia, 23
Herpetiform ulcers, mouth, 21
Hiatus hernia and oesophageal reflux, 37
  para-oesophageal (rolling), 37
Hydrocortisone pellets in aphthous ulceration, 21
Hyperkeratosis, bite, 31–32

Immunosuppression and oral ulceration, 21, 22
Isosorbide in achalasia of the cardia, 52
Isotope emptying study in achalasia of the cardia, 52

Jaundice, conditions causing, 15

Keratosis, smoker's, 29

Leukaemia, oral ulceration, 26
Leukoplakia, 28
Lichen planus, mouth, 24
  causing plaque, 29
  management, 24
Life expectancy, 8–9
Lips
  in Behçet's syndrome, 26, 27
  carcinoma, 34
  Herpes zoster, 23
Liver disorders, 15
Longevity and life expectancy, 8–9
Lupus erythematosus causing plaque, 29
Lymphoma, malignant, mouth, 34

Macroglossia, 33
Manometry, oesophageal, in achalasia of the cardia, 52
Metals, heavy, poisoning, oral ulceration, 27
Metronidazole in acute ulcerative gingivitis, 21
Motility disorders, oesophagus, 49–55
Mouth, diseases, 20–35
  see also Oral and specific names
Mucosal changes
  duodenum, 72–74
    bulbar duodenitis, 73
    coeliac disease, 72
    duodenitis and achlorhydria, 73

INDEX

and pernicious anaemia, 73
  villous atrophy, 73
  in gastritis, 59
  protection in ulcer, 65, 66, 67

Neuralgia, post-herpetic, 23
Neutropenia, chronic, oral ulceration, 26
Nifedipine, in achalasia of the cardia, 52
  in diffuse oesophageal spasm, 54
Non-steroidal anti-inflammatory drugs, and oesophagitis, 42
  and peptic ulcer disease, 66, 69
Nutrition and the elderly, 15
  and senile dementia, 15
Nystatin, in infective oesophagitis, 43–44
  in oral candidiasis, 22

Oesophagitis, infective, 43–44
  investigations, 43
  treatment, 43–44
Odynophagia, 43, 44
Oesophageal carcinoma, 45–49
  incidence, 45
  management, 47–49
  symptoms, 46
  types, 46–47
Oesophageal disease, elderly, 36–57
Oesophageal reflux, 36–57
  advice sheet, 39
  barium meal, 36–38
  complications, 40–42
  endoscopy, 38
  investigations, 36–37
  management, 38–40
  symptoms, 36
Oesophageal spasm, diffuse, 53–54
  see also Diffuse oesophageal spasm
Oesophagitis, drug-induced, 42–43
Oesophagus, motility disorders, 49–55
Oral carcinoma, 22–23
Oral tumours, 33–35
  carcinoma, 34
  management, 34–35
  pseudotumours, 33–35
  spread, 34–35
Oral ulceration, 20–23
  cause, 20
  drug-induced, 21
  resulting from trauma, 22
  and systemic disease, 26–27
  see also Mouth: specific disorders
Oropharyngeal dysphagia, 49

Palate
  hard, ulcers, 21
  soft, ulcers, 21
Pemphigoid, oral, 25
Pemphigus, oral, 26
Penicillin in acute ulcerative gingivitis, 21
Peptic stricture complicating oesophageal reflux, 40–42
  barium x-ray, 40
Peptic ulcer disease, pathogenesis, 66
  see also Duodenal ulcer: Gastric ulcer
Pernicious anaemia, 62–63
  cancer risk, 62–63
  and duodenitis, 73
  endoscopy, 73
  latent/manifest, 62
  gastric dysplasia, 63
Pharyngeal pouch, 50
  average age, 50
  barium swallow, 49
  contraindicating endoscopy, 11
  investigations, 50
  treatment, 50
Pigmentation, oral, 30
Pneumatic dilatation in diffuse oesophageal spasm, 53, 54
Polypectomy, 17
  perforation and bleeding, 17
Polyps
  cauterization, 17
  electrocoagulation, 17
  polypectomy, 17
Population changes
  since 1850, 8–9
  1986–2001, 9
Progressive systemic sclerosis, 54–55
Pseudotumours, oral, 33–35

Raynaud's phenomenon, 55
Renal disease, oral ulceration, 26

Saliva, artificial, 31
Scar, duodenal, endoscopy, 12
Sialorrhoea, 31
Sjögren's syndrome, xerostomia, 30
Smoker's keratosis, 29
Squamous carcinoma, oesophagus, 44, 46, 47
Steroids in
  Behçet's syndrome, 26
  oral erythema multiforme, 24–25
  oral lichen planus, 24
  oral pemphigoid, 25
Stomach
  ageing, 13–14, 58–64

mucosal changes, 58
  biopsy investigations, 59
Stomatitis
  denture, 22
  in renal disease, 26
Swallowing see Dysphagia
Syphilis and oral ulceration, 23
Systemic sclerosis, progressive, 54–55

Taste, disturbance, 32
Tetracycline mixture for aphthous ulceration, 21
Tongue
  abnormalities, 32
  carcinoma, 22, 34
  geographic, 32
  Herpes zoster, 23
  lichen planus and *Candida*, 25
  pigmentation, 30
Treatable illness in old age, 10
Treatment
  techniques, 13
  see also specific therapy
Triamcinolone acetonide in aphthous ulcers, 21
Tuberculosis and oral ulceration, 23
Tumours see special names, origins or regions

Ulceration, oral, 20–23
  causes, 20
  see also specific disorders

Vesicles, oral, 30–32
Villous atrophy in duodenitis, 73
Vitamin B_{12} deficiency, 62, 63
  causes, 62, 63
  oral ulceration, 26

Wegener's granulomatosis, oral ulceration, 27
Weight loss, 15
  and senile dementia, 15

Xerostomia, 31
  characteristics, 31

Zenker's diverticulum see Pharyngeal pouch
Zinc chloride mouthwash for aphthous ulceration, 21
Zollinger-Ellison syndrome, 68